also by nicklaus suino

Budo Mind and Body: Training Secrets of the Japanese Martial Arts (comprehensive revision of *Arts of Strength, Arts of Serenity*)

Arts of Strength, Arts of Serenity

Strategy in Japanese Swordsmanship

Practice Drills for Japanese Swordsmanship

The Art of Japanese Swordsmanship

Look Up!

The Drinking Game

101 Ideas to Kick Your Ass Into Gear (with Ian A. Gray)

Success Sandbox: A Development Journal of Success & Happiness (with Ian A. Gray)

SEO and Beyond: How to Rocket Your Website to Page One of Google! (with Don E. Prior III)

the flywheel

for humble
mother truckers
who want to
hit really
really
hard

the flywheel

for humble mother truckers who want to hit really really hard

nicklaus suino

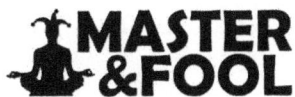

MASTER &FOOL

Master and Fool, LLC
2875 Boardwalk, Suite H
Ann Arbor, Michigan 48104

10 9 8 7 6 5 4 3 2 1

FIRST EDITION

Written, Edited, and Printed in the
United States of America

ISBN: 978-0-578-74972-3

"Whether you're rich or poor,
it's nice to be able to hit really, really hard."
– Thomas Jefferson

contents

acknowledgements

I've been blessed with a few extraordinary teachers and a few exceptional training partners. This book brings together into one simple approach the key concepts they used to generate more power than you can believe a single human being is capable of dishing out.

All credit goes to them for the useful and the profound in this manual. All the errors and omissions are mine. These rock-stars helped make *The Flywheel* a reality. If I forgot anybody, it's because I've been hit in the head by a lot of tough people.

John "Doc" Spears
Nobetsu Tadanori
Gary Legacy
Tabata-Sensei ("Yoda")
John B. Gage
Sato Nobuyuki
Randy Dauphin
Satoh Tadayuki
Daniel Holland
Sato Shizuya

introduction
by John "Doc" Spears

One of the things that enriched my life happened when I finally came to the realization that there was simply not one best way of doing most anything. Even when our task is something as relatively straight forward as delivering an effective strike, the multitude of effective ways of doing so is humbling to consider.

Of course, for the student you must first learn a single correct way of doing something before you can consider the multitude of ways, lest you end up with a dozen ways to do something poorly. In martial skill, that's a recipe for self-delusion and disaster.

Once you gain competence, it's time to learn ways to improve your technique–even accepting there are methods radically different than those you were taught in your first martial training (you know, the one your first teacher told you was going to devastate an opponent, and you do it this way and no other, or it's wrong.)

And when you see a different way of doing it, a better way, now it is either an opportunity for growth, or an experience in ego deflation.

The mantra of dogma is always, "but this is how I was taught." When our goal is power, the punch is the truth, and nothing else. Either what you're doing is effective, or it isn't. The chains the heavy bag hangs from sing when you hit it, or they don't. Your partner tells you to ease back because his hand holding the mitt is numb, or it isn't. Your partner holding the air shield has to give up his stance with your roundhouse kick, or you bounce off it.

For those who take the path to learn beyond dogma, it becomes possible to develop a variety of tools in your toolbox of skills, ready for access on demand.

To folks like Nick Suino who've dedicated their lives to studying a tremendous variety of martial arts, that realization of the "different but same, same but different" came a lot sooner than it did to the rest of us.

The beauty of having such a diverse body of training and teaching as Nick is this; he learned early that it's the similarities rather than the dissimilarities between the different martial arts that matter. They're all practiced by the same human form. Styles, appearances, and distracting ostensible like uniforms sometimes cloud the basic truths of how our bodies are used most efficiently. Whether wielding a sword or using fists and feet, power comes from the same source. And it's the practitioner's goal to learn how to efficiently draw on that source.

The Flywheel is one of those. Nick's provided a great guide to help you to practice and most importantly, to think.

Training with a partner is ideal. Training tools like striking mitts and air shields will allow you to improve your mechanics and you and your partner will be able to feel the improvement in your power delivery. The heavy bag is an indispensable tool as well, but be careful!

For everyone there comes a day when too much power delivered to dense objects comes back to you as injury. Put variety in your training and avoid overuse.

Conditioning the parts of your body for striking is important. For your fists, knuckle push-ups on wood and concrete, striking the makiwara and the wooden dummy, and learning how to break blocks and boards are all important to get those surfaces ready for a fight. But such training doesn't make you impervious.

Funny thing about a fight; your opponent gets a say. He likes to move, too. That beautiful punch directed with the perfect rotation and follow through at your opponent's jaw suddenly lands on his dipped cranium. Instead of contacting with your perfectly conditioned first two knuckles, your third and fourth meet his skull. It's happened to me. It only took me a few broken bones to put into practice what I'd been told by smarter, older fighters. "Use a hard part of your body against a soft target, and a soft part of your body against a hard target." Heads are hard. And irregular, too. Nick shows you the open palm. Use it!

Martial arts are a discipline. And discipline is worth-while for its own sake. It makes you a better person. Whatever your goal in training is, I hope that under-standing striking power is at least one of those goals. Or else, we really are just waving our hands in the air.

– Doc

read this first

The concepts in this book can help you hit a lot harder.

If you do the work, you'll make the person holding the focus mitt gasp when you hit it. You may pop an air shield or break a heavy bag in half. In self-defense (don't pick fights) you could drop your attacker to the pavement like a cold side of beef. It could save your life.

Whether you're into self-defense, sparring or winning tournaments, it's good to know how to hit hard and hit fast with little effort, and how to do it while moving smoothly, maintaining your balance and exposing yourself to low risk.

Sounds too good to be true, I know.

There's no such thing as an easy path to greatness, but you can get there a lot faster with *The Flywheel*.

the flywheel

I've trained and taught martial arts for over 50 years throughout North America and Japan. I've competed in a ton of tournaments and won medals and high honors. I've done long spans in these styles:

- Goju-Ryu Karate
- Judo
- Nihon Jujutsu
- Iaido
- Kyudo
- Shorin-Ryu Karate
- Aikido
- San Chuan Dao

I've also attended seminars and paid close attention to experts in widely varied styles like these:

- Shotokan Karate
- BJJ
- Hung-Gar Kung Fu
- Hsing-I and Bagua
- Tai Chi
- Wrestling
- Boxing

I've learned a lot about the combat arts, usually the hard way. I wrote this book for two reasons:

1. There are **universal principles of movement** that show up in all important fighting disciplines; and

2. **People make a lot of mistakes**. Those mistakes rob them of power, slow them down, expose them to risk, and cause acute and chronic injuries.

The Flywheel is a simple striking system based on key principles. It helps eliminate many common mistakes. It will give you tools to strike harder and faster with less effort while moving smoothly, maintaining your balance and exposing yourself to less risk. You can:

- stay fit with a few hours a week on the heavy bag.
- get better at self-defense.
- amplify your power for karate, kick-boxing, Muay Thai, or whatever you train.
- raise your game for sparring or ring fighting.

Don't be stupid and get into bar fights or street fights. Even so-called "winners" in brawls, bare knuckle contests and boxing matches get injured and risk brain damage. You may also wind up in court, where your reputation, your money, and your freedom are at risk.

Having said all that, being able to punch and kick really, really hard is good, clean fun. Let's get started!

chapter one

flywheel theory

flywheel | ʻfli (h)wel | - noun
a heavy revolving wheel in a machine that
increases momentum and provides a reserve of power to
drop on a dumbass who messes with you.

That's the secret of *The Flywheel* – to increase momentum
and provide a reserve of power. The better job you do, the
faster and more powerful your strikes will be. Think about
the flywheel when you're building your chain of power.

This isn't a tactical book and you probably wouldn't understand
it if it was, so don't focus on the good looking dude in the
pictures – he's just there to help you lunkheads understand
the big words.

Look at the way the hips are supposed to move and learn
from it. Do the moves big at first to feel your potential power.
Later, as your body and mind start to come together, refine the
techniques and wire them into whatever hairbrained fighting
system you already use.

flywheel theory part one
- the hip is the flywheel

Think of your pelvis as a flywheel. Learn to move it in a horizontal circle first. Later you can tilt the circle to deliver power at upward and downward angles.

Look at the picture on page 3. That arrow shows how the hip should rotate, like the agitator in your Mom's washing machine. If you did your own laundry once in a while, you'd understand this better.

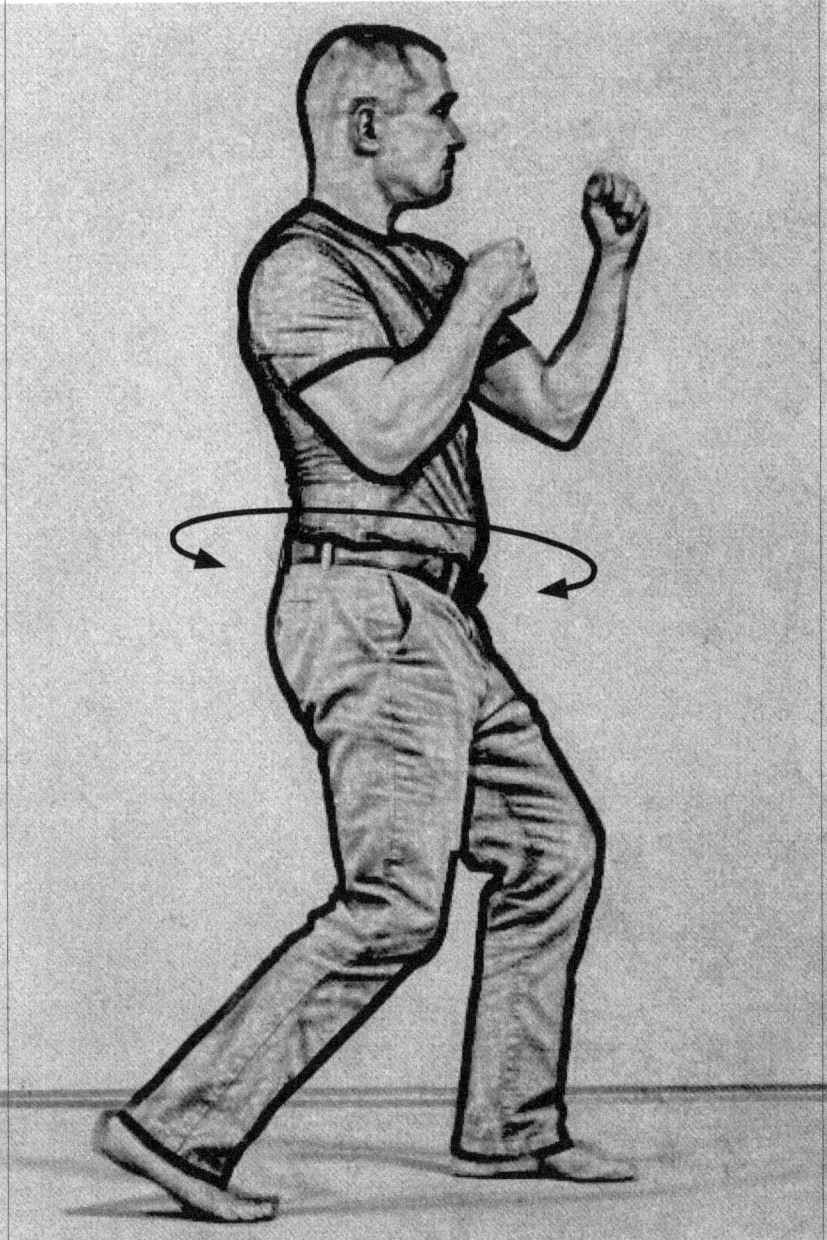

flywheel theory part two
- the ball of the back foot
is a key power source

If you're as old as I am, you remember when people used to smoke cigarettes in public.

They'd drop their cigarette butt on the ground and smash it with their foot. They'd grind it out by circling their foot back and forth. Try that motion.

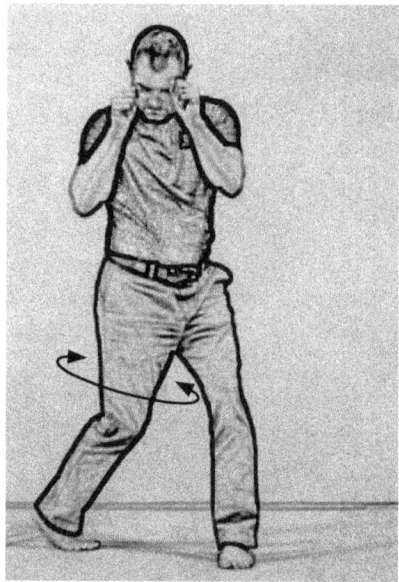

Put your left foot forward and keep most of your weight on it. Pivot the ball of your right foot on the floor so your heel moves in a horizontal arc.

You power a lot of flywheel moves with the ball of the back foot. Learn to rotate it to: (a) *allow* the hip to turn freely; and (2) *power* the hip turn.

Page 5 is shows you another view of how to turn your hip and heel for flywheel power. Stay in school, kids!

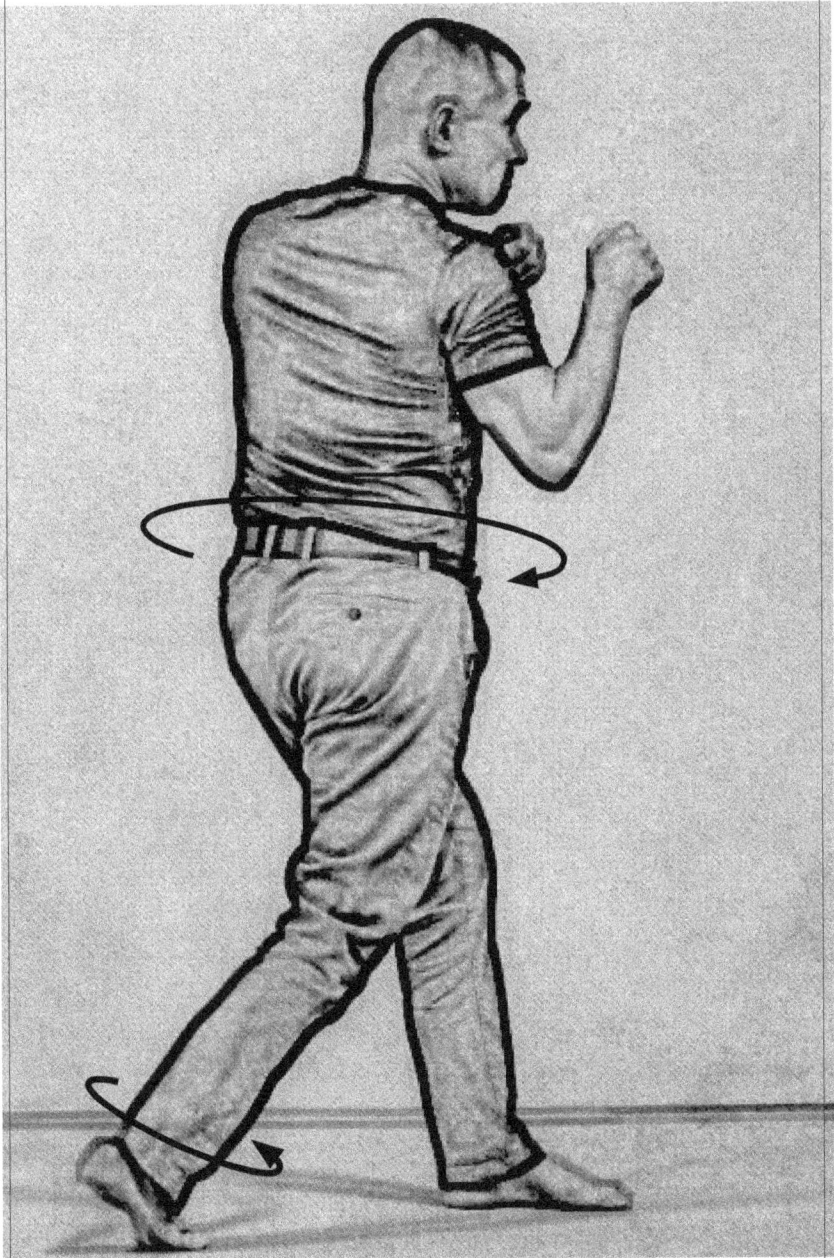

corollary to part one
- a flat back foot can work against you

Take note that a flat back foot can work against you. If you leave it behind, there's none of the power benefit you get from the ball of the foot. You can work up *some* hip power, but can also get stretched out and lose the ability to recover your balance quickly.

Look at how the back foot appears stuck in this picture and how the hip rotation is limited.

In the picture on page 7, the hips have been pushed forward by a strong back foot and leg. That shows how you get linear strength.

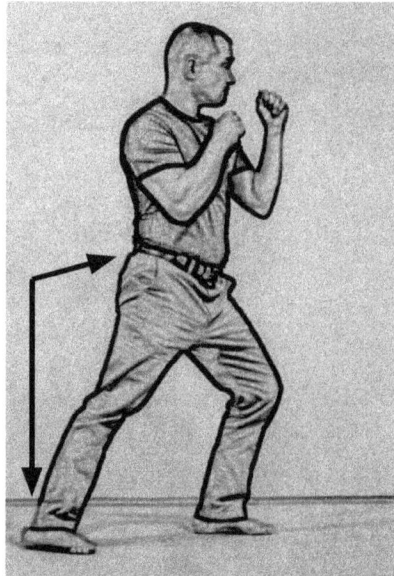

You could drive that power into a jab or a front-leg front kick, or follow up with a right cross. But settle down, Skippy ... let's learn how to move well before you get fancy.

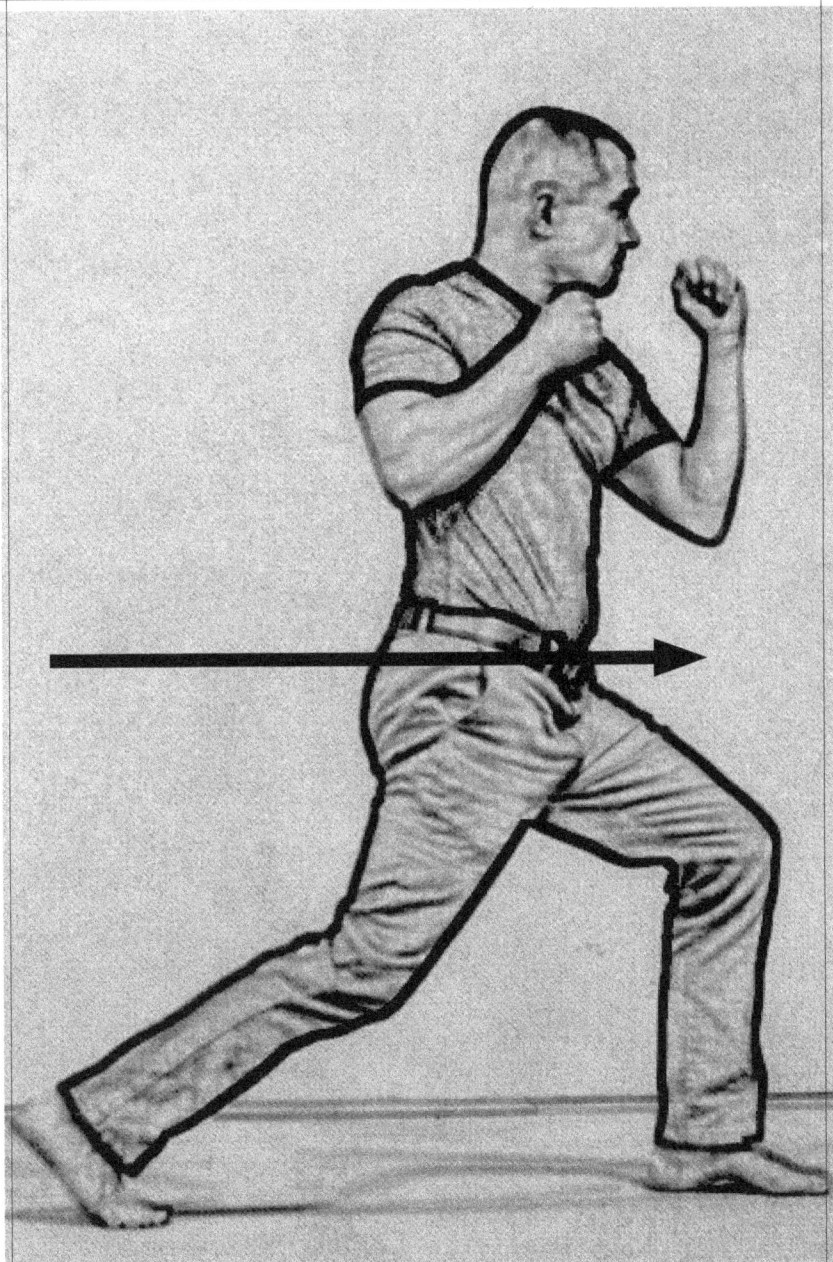

flywheel theory part three
- a solid base leg supports the flywheel

For great balance and great power, you need a strong base. That base is usually the front leg. The core components of the base leg are:

- Foot straight ahead.
- Knee bent
- Knee aligned with the centerline of the foot.
- Most of the bodyweight on the front leg.
- Ability to rotate the hip without moving the knee.

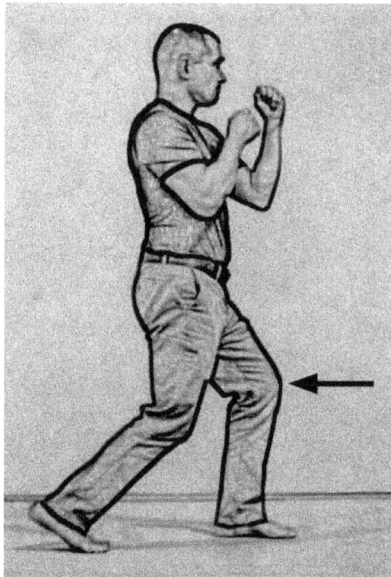

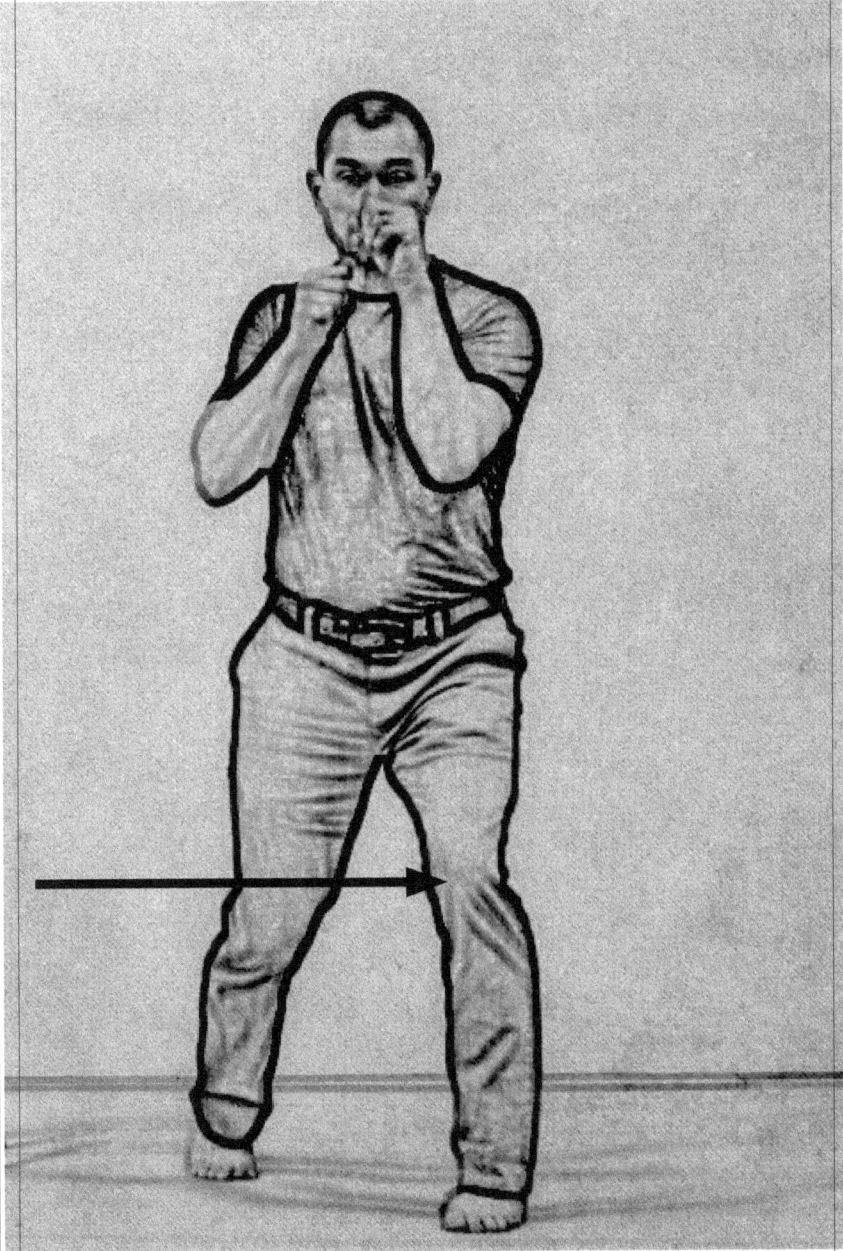

flywheel theory part four
- rotate the flywheel to drive strikes

The hip throws punches straight out, then pulls the arm straight back.

The picture below shows the flywheel driving the right arm straight out.

The picture on page 11 shows the flywheel throwing a circular, open-hand strike out. The arm would rotate back as you return to the compact guard position.

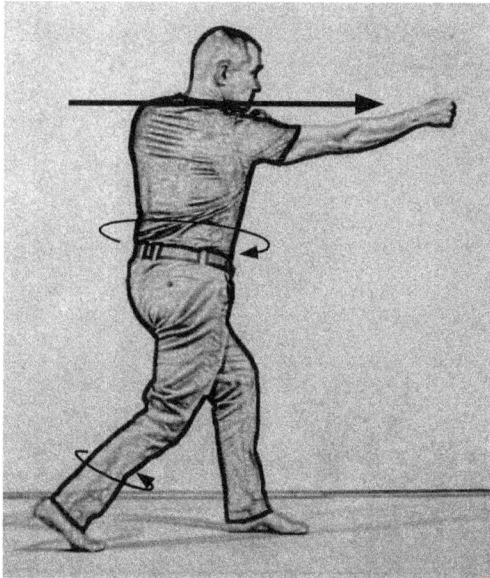

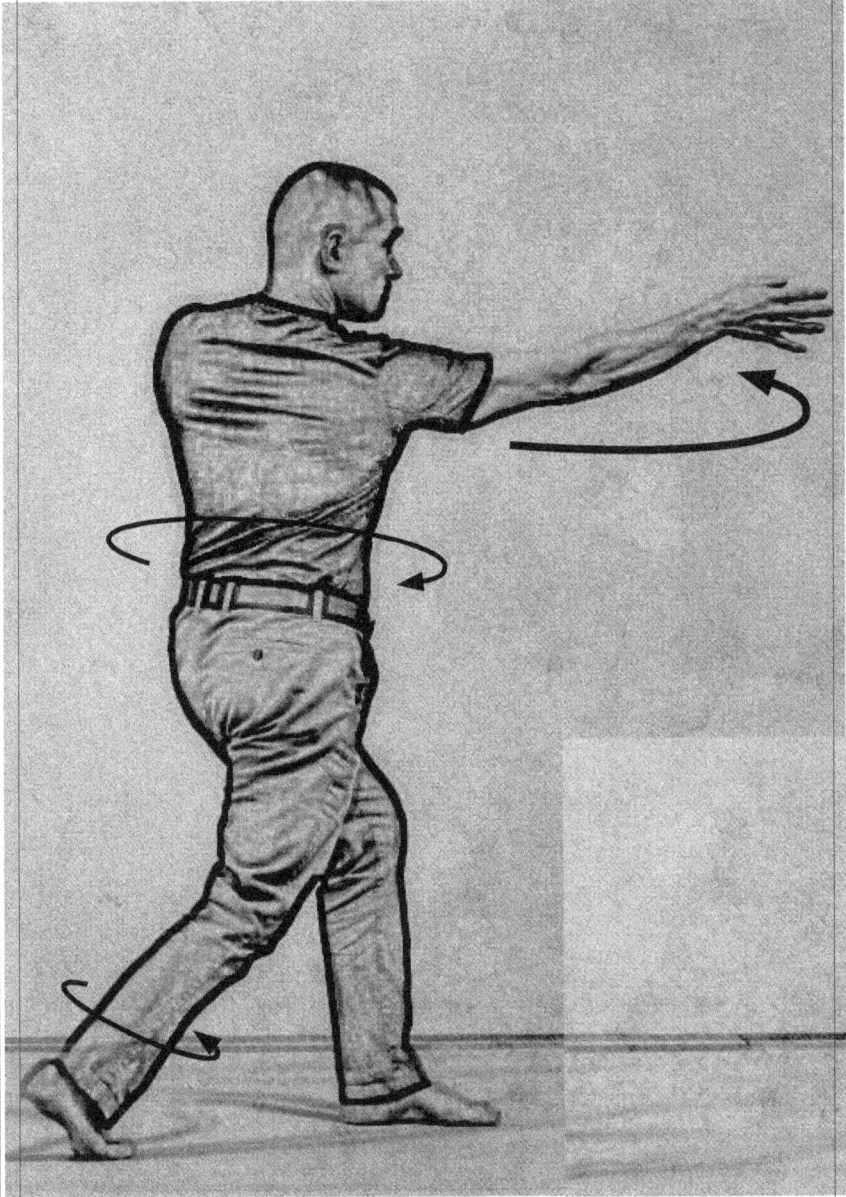

flywheel theory part four
- return to guard

Always complete the circles. Make it a habit to return to a compact, balanced, relaxed guard position. That will help you get more natural power, stay in better balance, cover up against counterstrikes, and be ready to move explosively again.

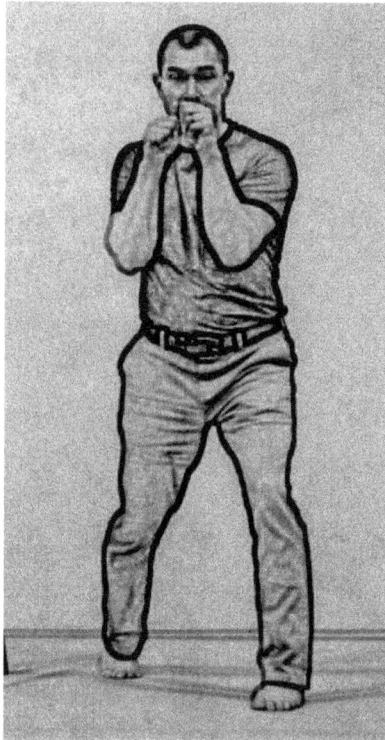

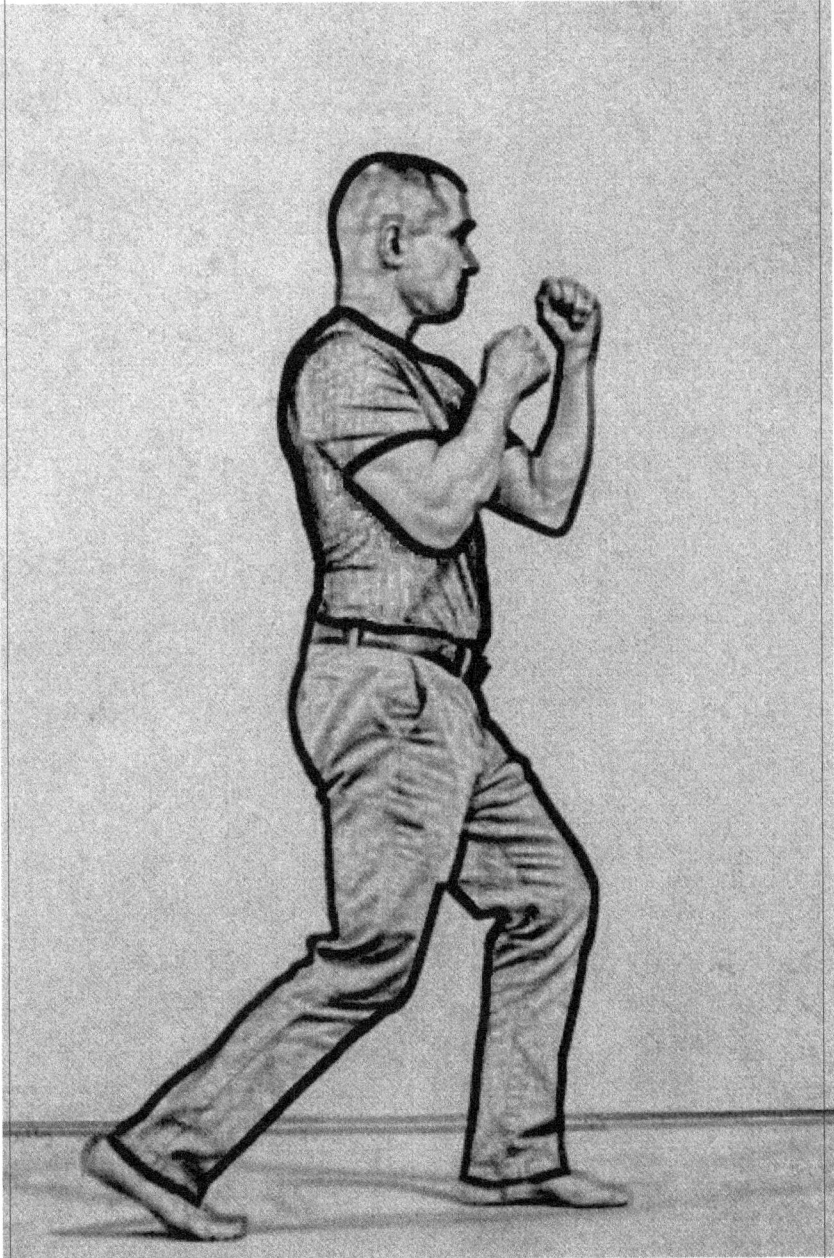

the flywheel

flywheel notes
1. turn only on one leg - not both

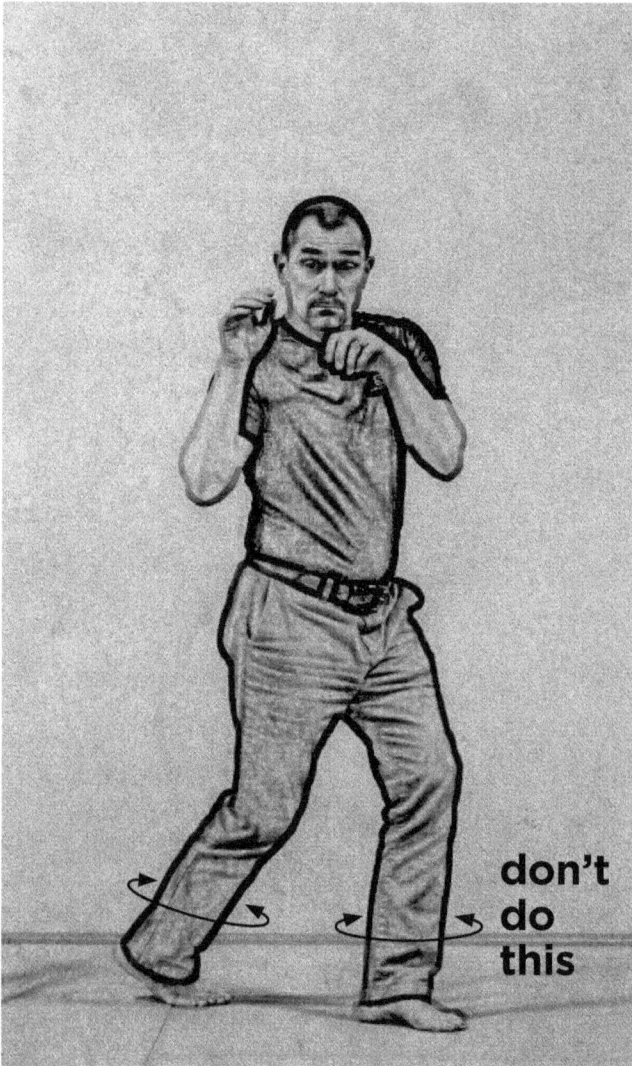

don't
do
this

2. rotate on the ball of the back foot like there's a spike through it

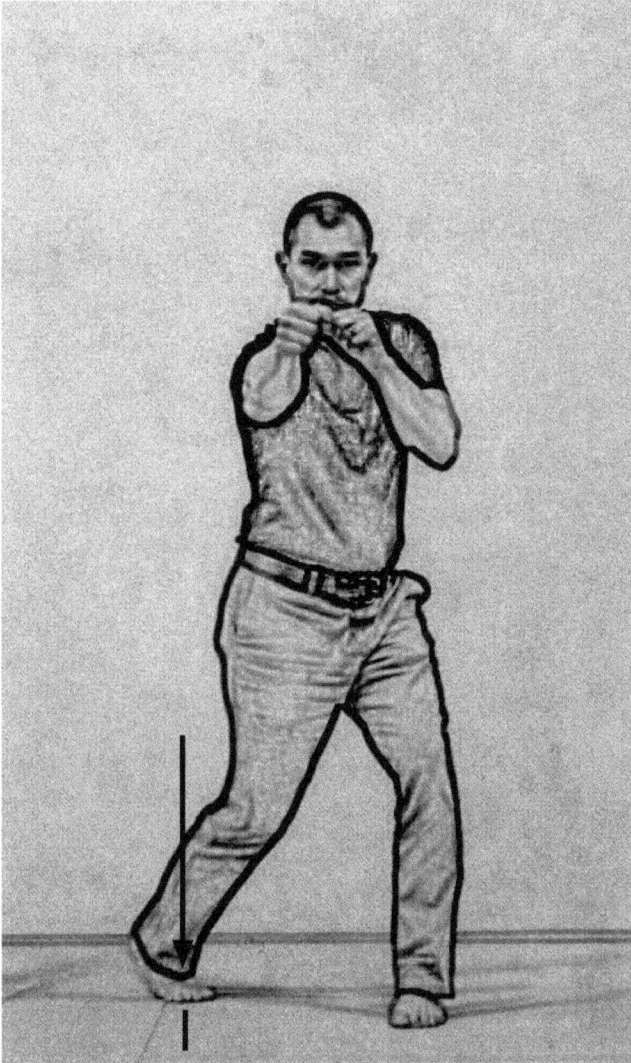

3. keep the base leg knee slightly bent and aligned over the lead foot

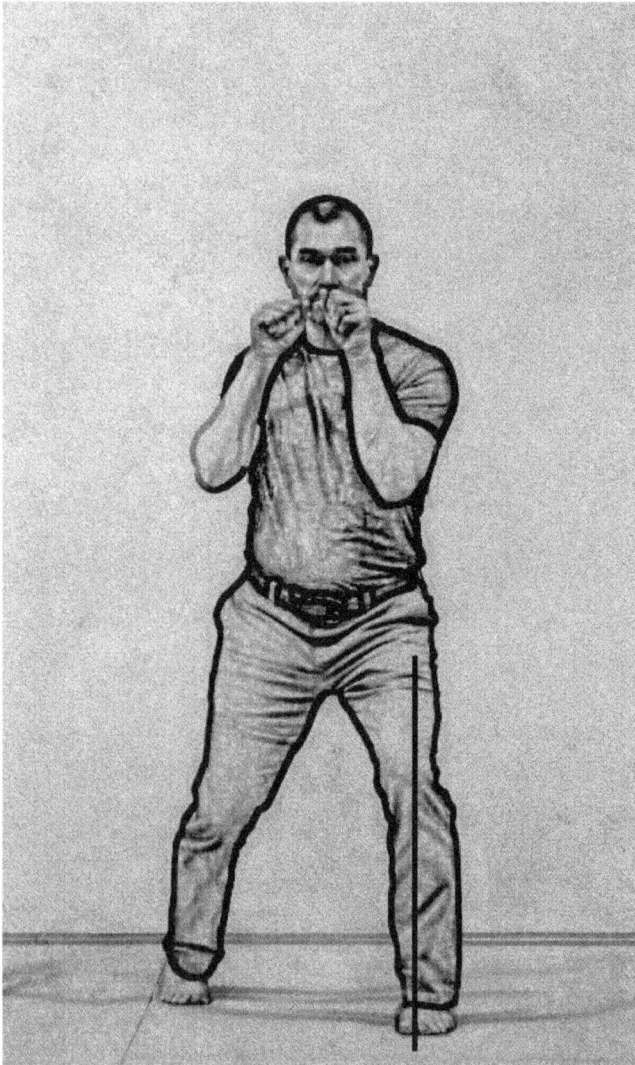

4. keep some width between the feet for balance

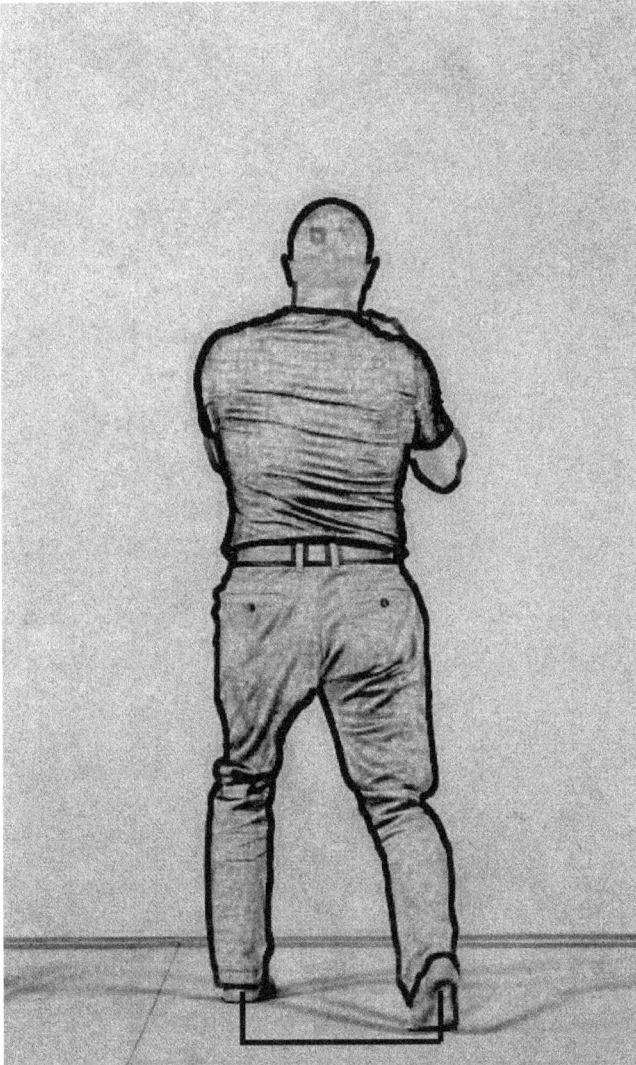

the flywheel

5. get very good at turning the hips

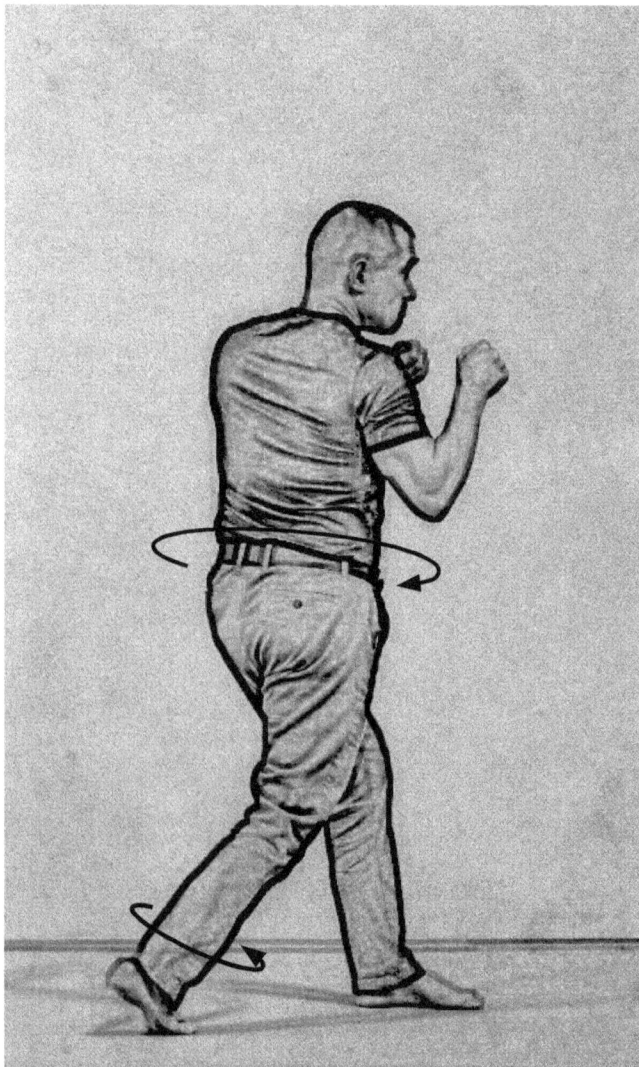

6. practice stepping with the lead leg, then planting the ball of the back foot

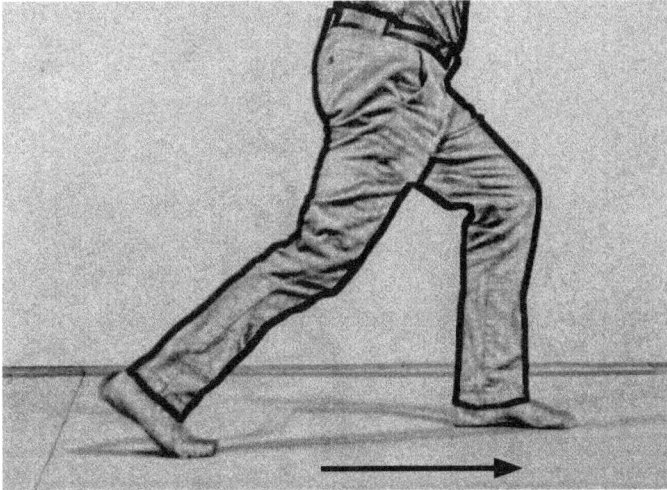

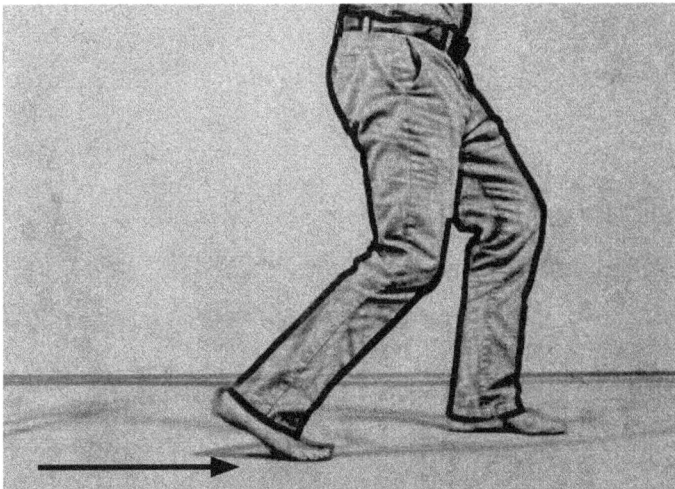

chapter two

relaxation strikes

"Just chill, homie." - Sir Isaac Newton

Being able to relax is your key to fast, effortless movement. Most people and even many accomplished fighters are terrible at relaxing when the pressure's on.

You should practice relaxing outside of training to develop the skillset. There are a million ways to do that, including things like:

- Meditation
- Breathing
- Yoga
- Dance lessons
- Judo grappling or BJJ
- Wearing sexy underwear
- Pretending you're a Jeep

On the next few pages you'll see key tools to relax your body and make your striking more powerful.

the flywheel

loose hand drop

Drop your open hand from overhead to a horizontal mitt. Keep your fingers back so your palm hits first, not your fingers. Work on this until you can let your arm drop without adding tension.

This is practice, not fighting, so success is measured by how well you relax, not how much effort you exert. Lighten up, Alice!

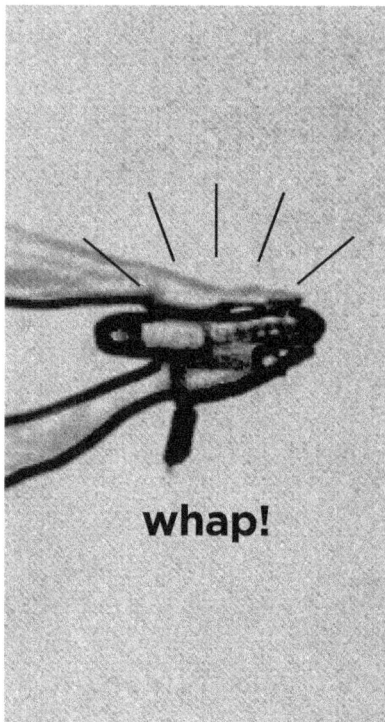

whap!

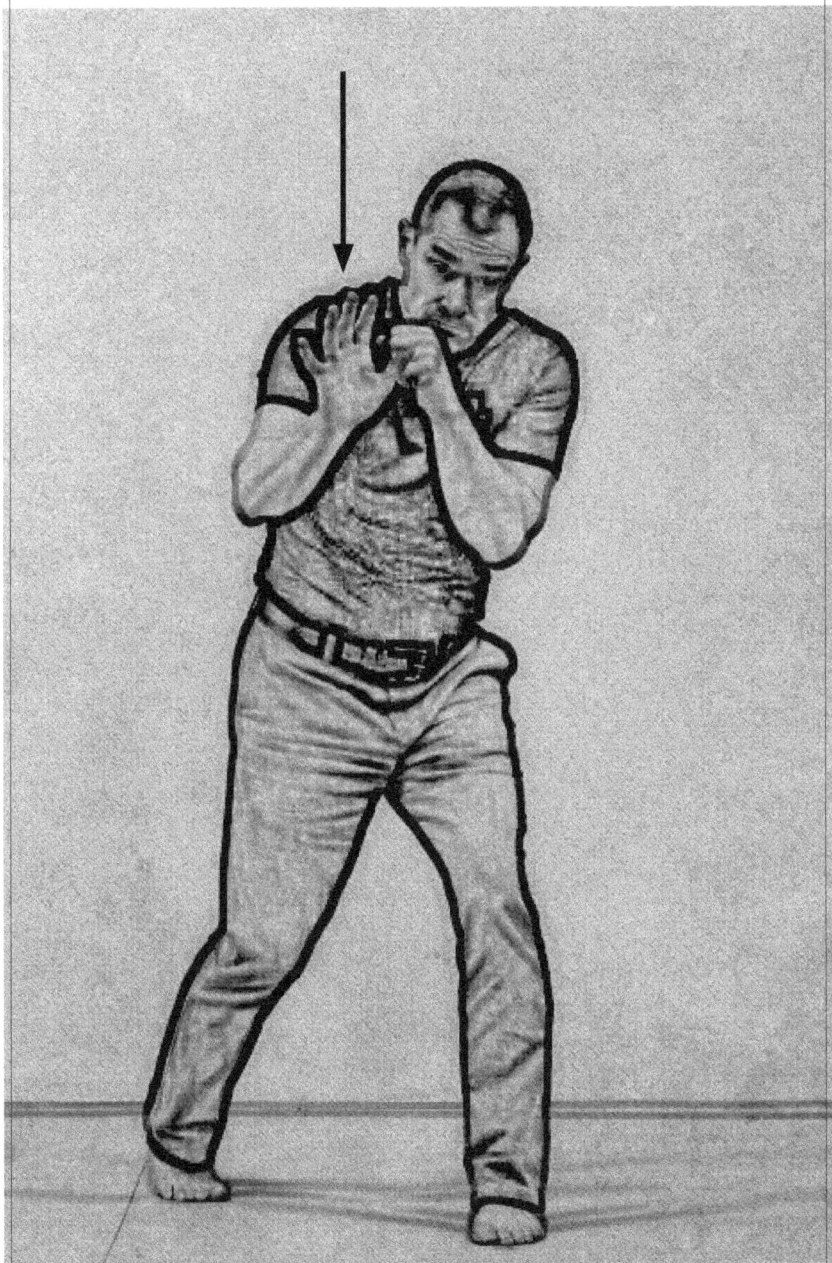

accelerated hand drop

Do what you just did ... drop your open hand from overhead to a horizontal mitt. But this time, accelerate your hand. Adjust your position until you can make a big "WHAP!"

Stay relaxed! Work at it until you have super hero power with little or no muscle tension.

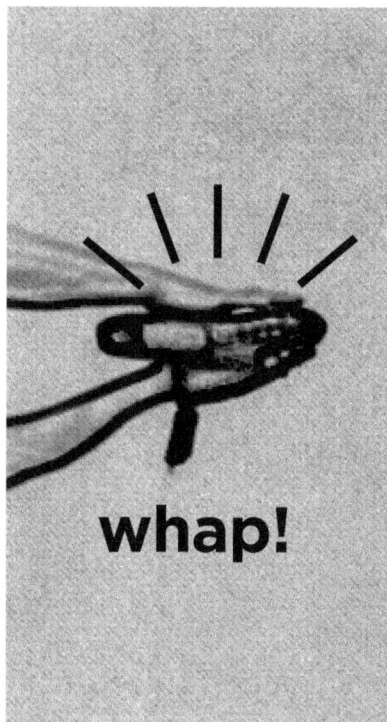

whap!

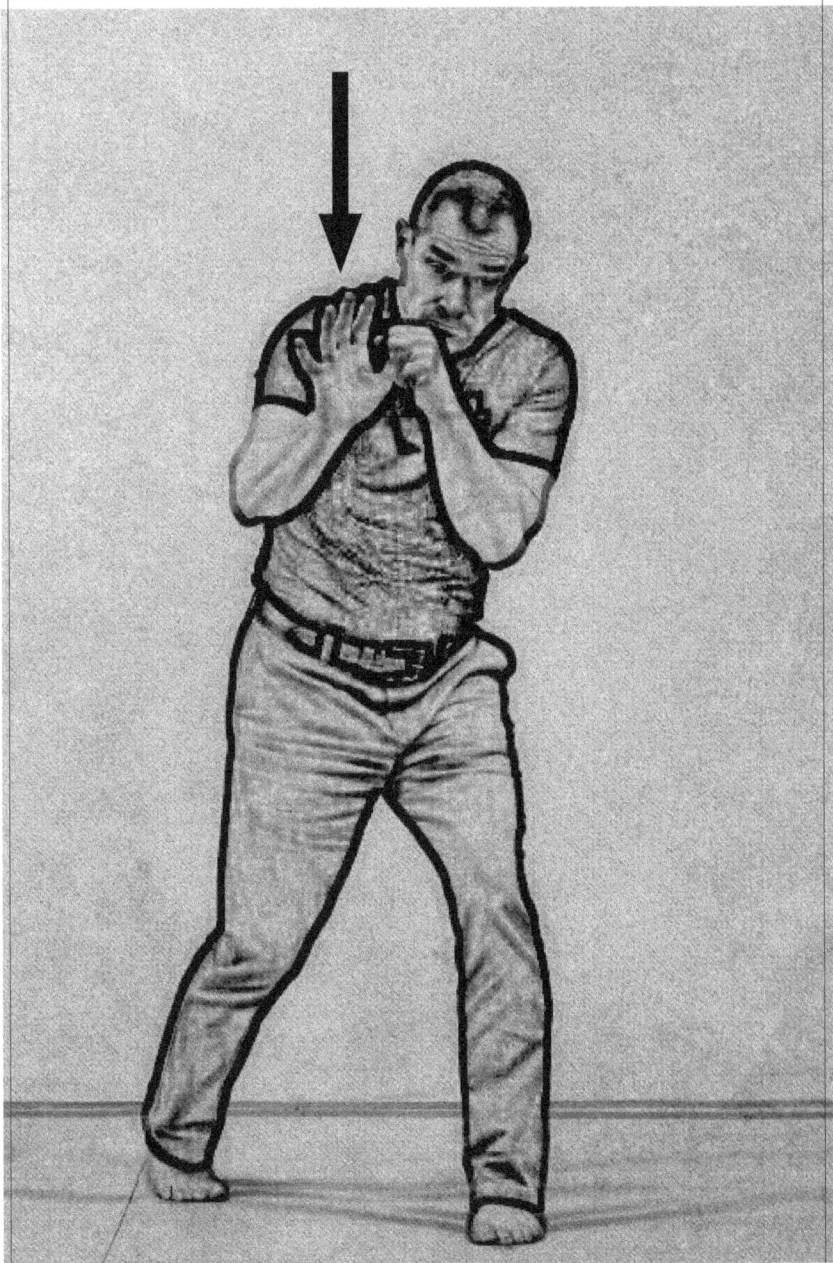

throw your hand out

Now have your partner hold the mitt at the level of your nose. Throw your hand at the mitt. Remember the feel of the first two relaxation strikes and try to maintain it.

Make the motion really big at first. Adjust your position until you can really generate a big "WHAP!"

You can tailor it for tactical use later – right now, try to be as loose as you can to get a ton of momentum without tensing your muscles. Keep your fingers back to ensure good contact with the palm of your hand.

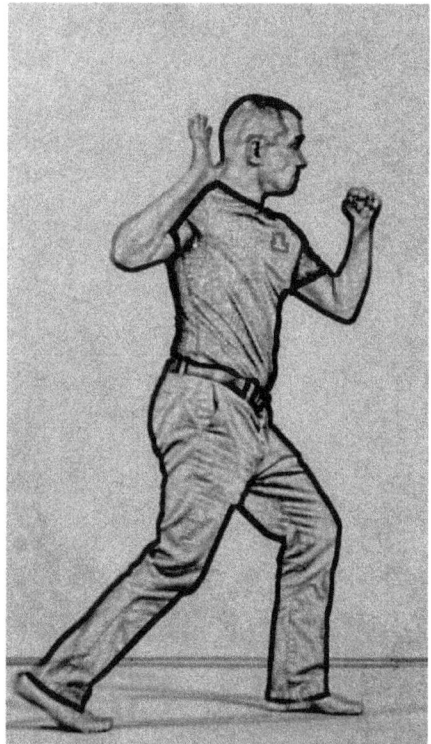

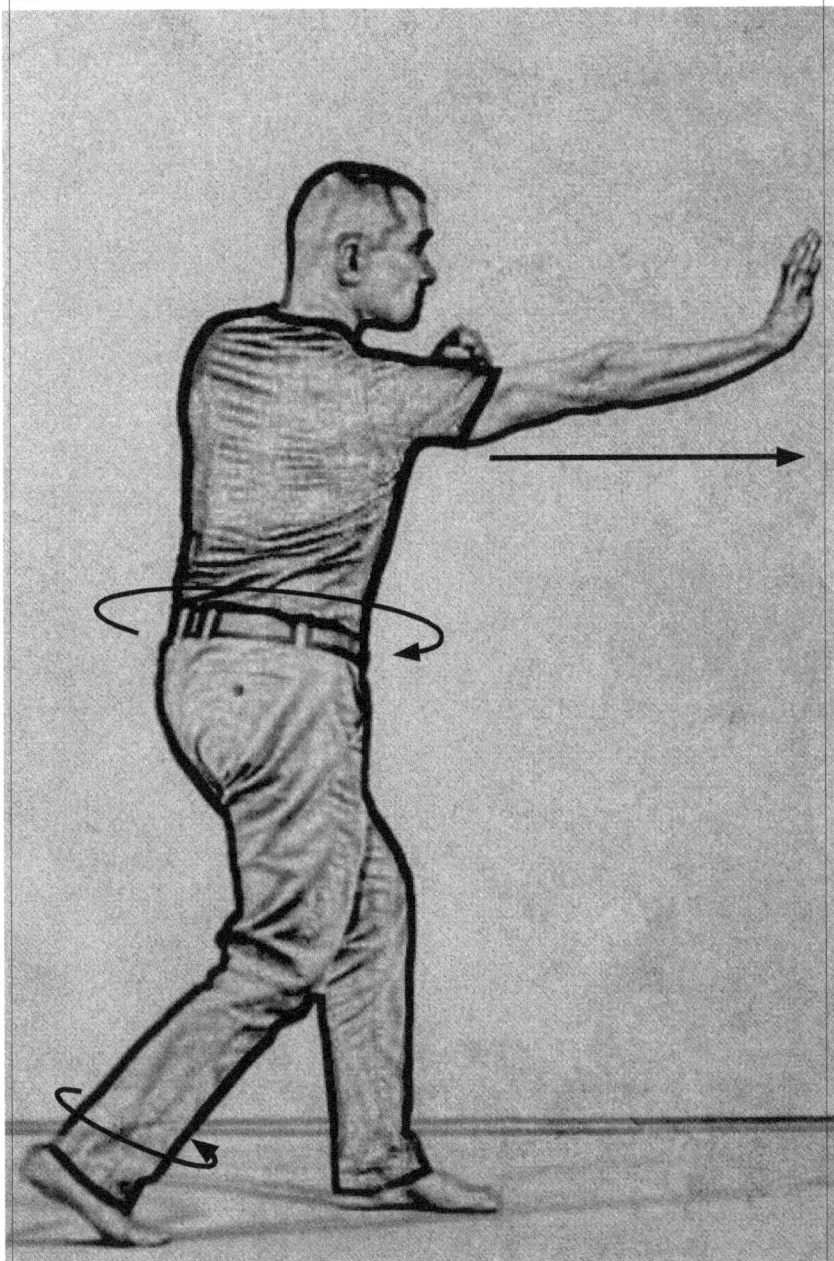

throw a punch out

Make sure you know how to make a good fist.

There's a section about fists starting on page 52. You're allowed to skip ahead and then come back here. Mom said it's okay, so go check on that, then come back here.

Once you get the feel for a good fist and relaxed shoulders, throw your hand at the mitt. Start light. A relaxed throw is a win right now, not a hard hit. Tune your position and your speed until you can hit the mitt really hard while staying relaxed.

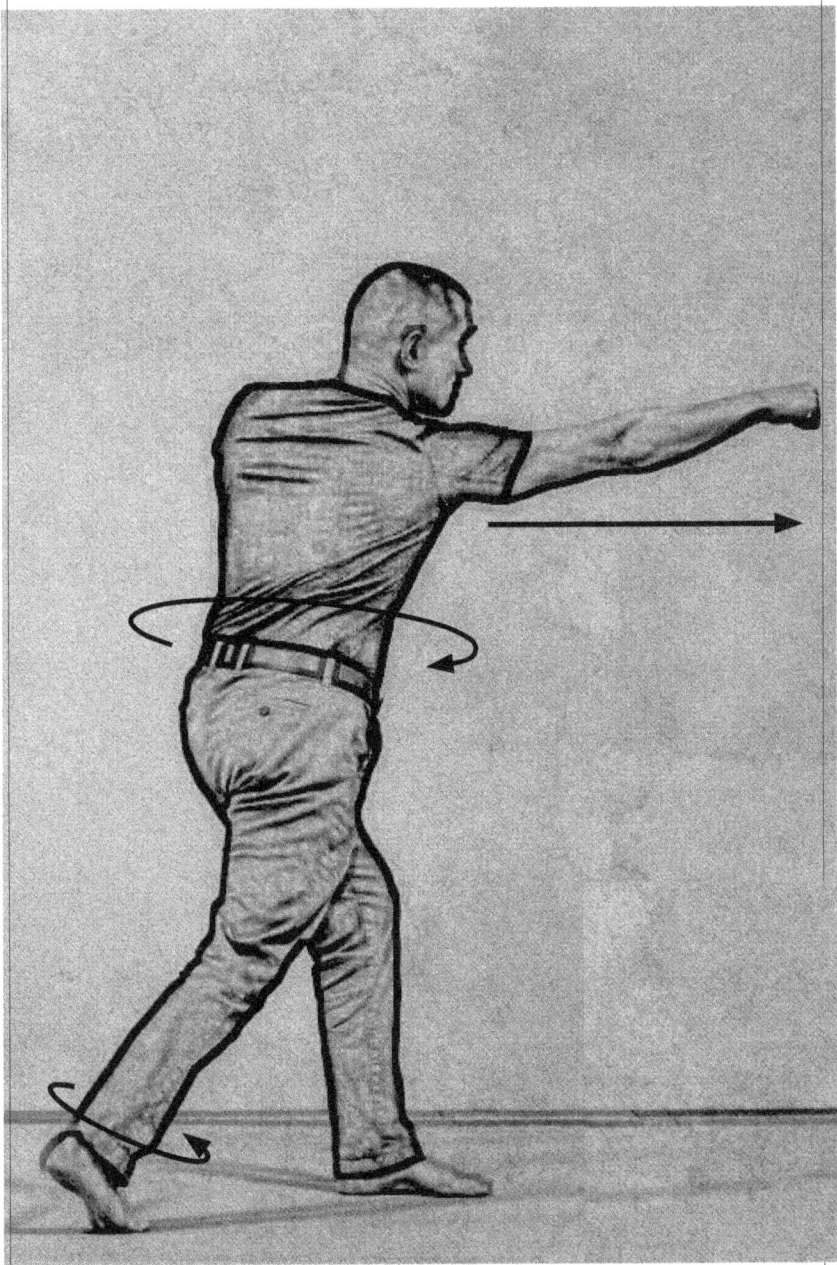

chapter three

holding focus mitts

"I hate jackwagons who don't know how to hold focus mitts." - Friedrich Nietzsche

Holding focus mitts properly is an underrated skill. Do it badly and your partner's training will suffer. They could even get injured.

Do it well and you'll not only keep your partner safer, they'll learn a lot faster!

Let them feel the heaviness of the strike, but don't drive the mitt into the striking hand ... save that for gloved practice.

align the face of the mitt
perpendicular to the path of the strike

Align the face of the mitt perpendicular to the path of the strike.

"Perpendicular" means at a right angle. Words too hard? Look at the pictures!

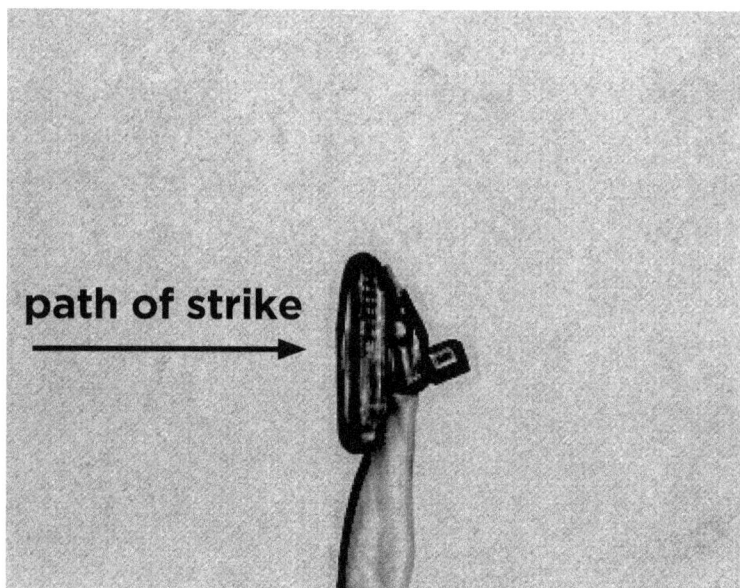

path of strike

watch your tilt!

Beginners screw this up all the time. You have to build awareness of the mitt position.

Tilting the top downward reduces felt power and increases the risk of knuckle and wrist injury.

Just stop it.

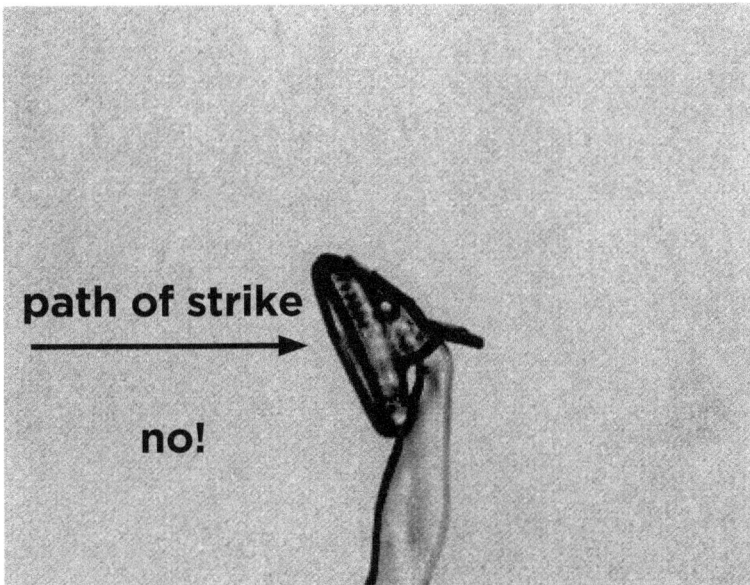

maintain a right angle in your shoulder

If your arm is straight out to the side, your shoulder has no room to open up. Hold the mitt at a right angle to your shoulder, especially for big power strikes. Then you can let your arm swing back if your training partner gets lucky enough to deal out a rare powerful strike.

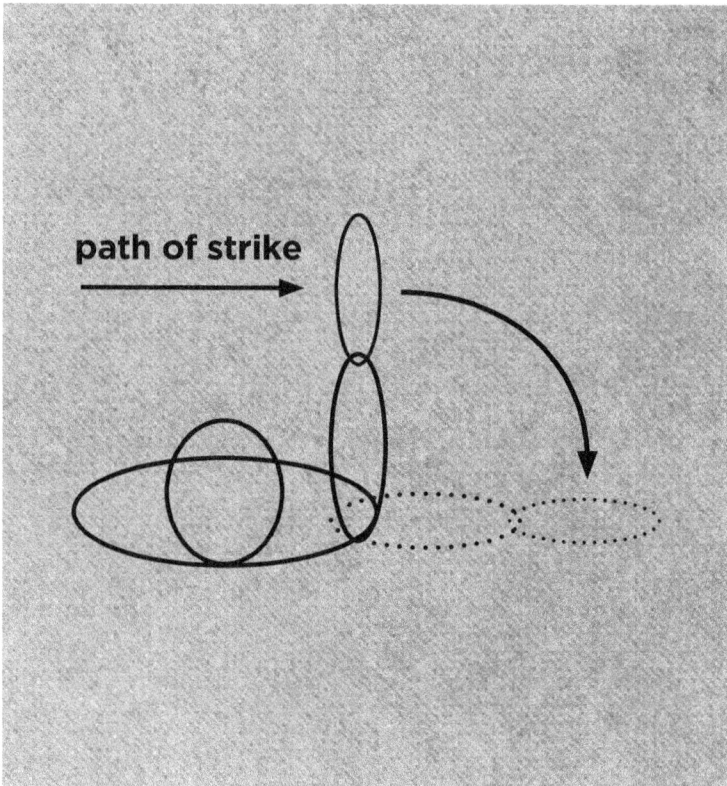

path of strike

when you hold one or two mitts close, puncher reduces power

For multiple punch drills, you'll hold two mitts. If you're holding them closer to your body or in a way that reduces your shoulder mobility, the puncher should reduce power.

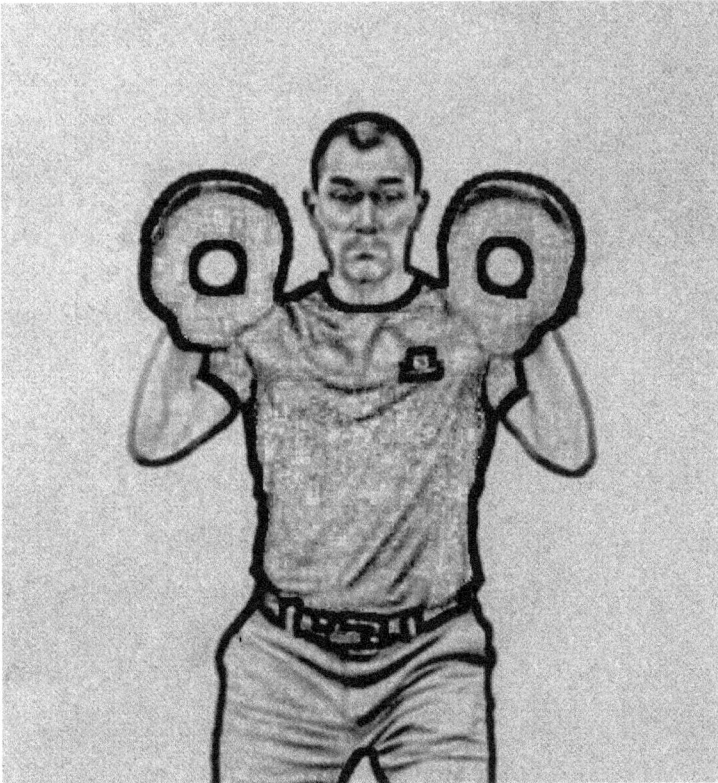

chapter four

open hand strikes

"When a throat punch doesn't work, just try smacking the dust off their smirking faces."
- Indira Ghandi

These open hand strikes are meant to let you practice while staying as relaxed as possible.

They are also useful for striking when you haven't built up your knuckles, don't want to draw blood, or want to hit somebody's hard brain casing without breaking your hand, like Doc said in the introduction.

I've seen amazing results when I've taught these to non-martial artists in self-defense classes, especially smaller, slightly built women who are shocked to realize how much power they can generate.

the flywheel

throw a jab

Throw a jab with an open hand. As with relaxation strikes, try to keep your fingers back so your palm hits the mitt first.

"Throw" means throw. Start big and loose until you get the feel for letting this rip. Later you can make it more compact and strategic.

The power for the jab comes from pushing the hip forward with ball of the foot power. There is a small hip circle. When you jab with the left hand as shown, the left hip moves forward first – powered by the right leg – then moves back as you reset to guard position.

Getting a fast, heavy jab is hard for a lot of people, but you can do hard things. The trick for simpletons like you and me is to just keep practicing and relax!

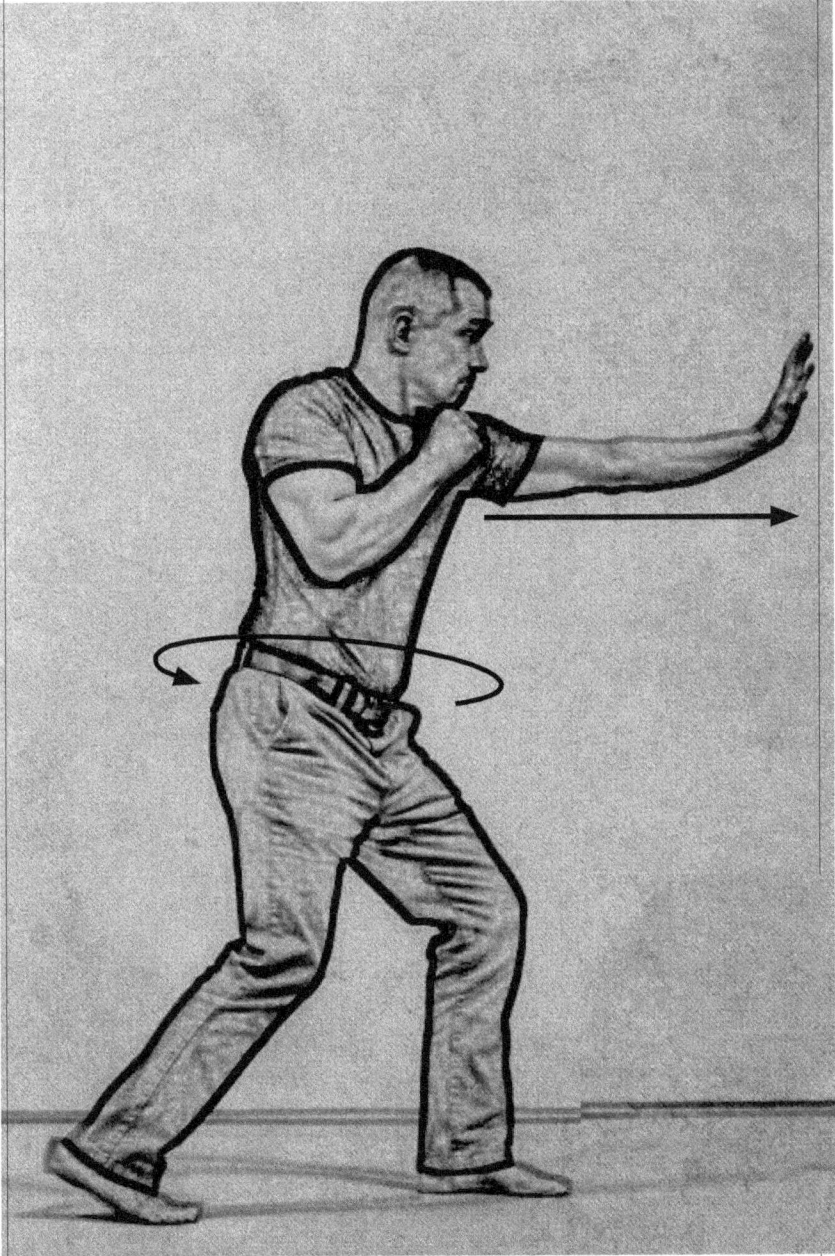

throw a cross

Throw a cross with an open hand. Turn the hip and heel to start the throw. Keep most of your weight on your base leg with your knee slightly bent.

The power for the cross comes from the flywheel. Press down with the ball of the back foot a micro-second before launching the strike. The hip circle is bigger than it is for the jab.

Always finish the circle. Reset to your compact guard position, in balance, ready to throw the next relaxed, heavy strike.

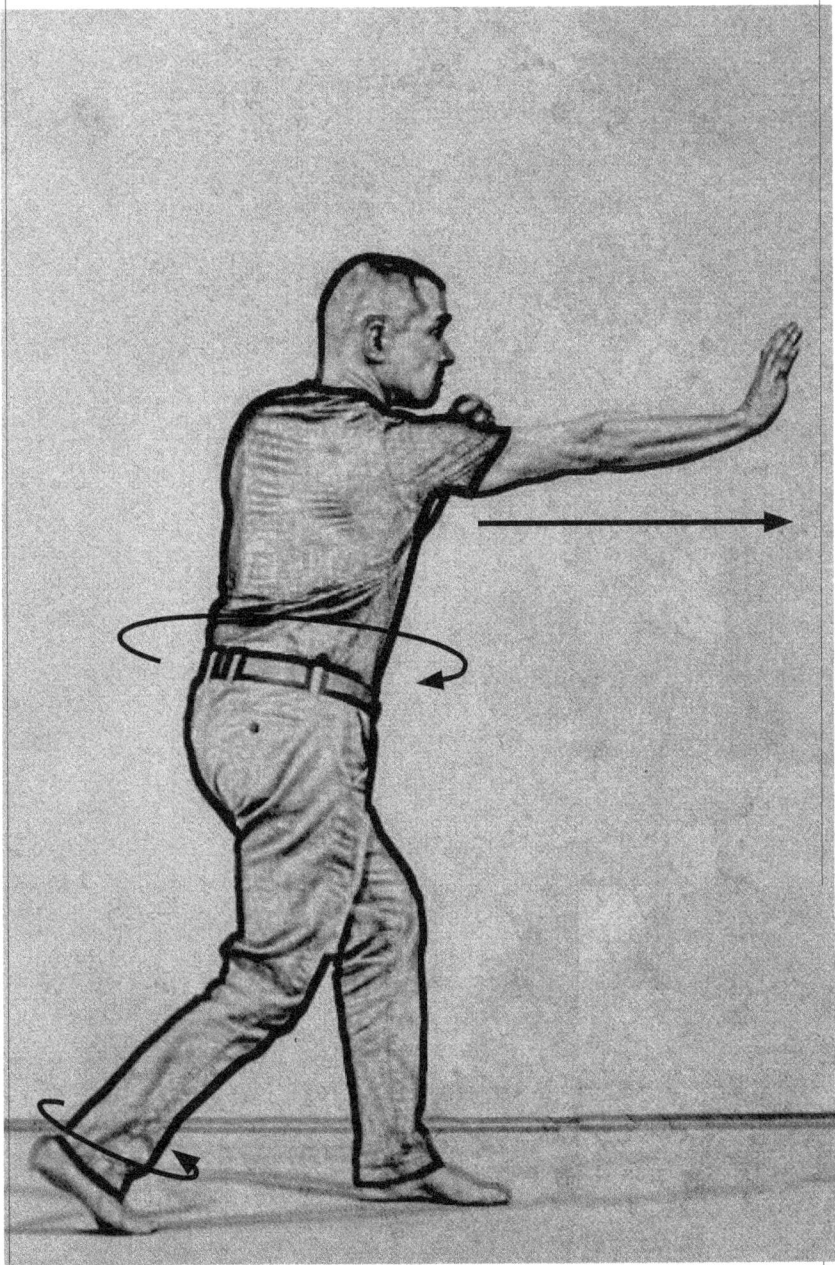

the flywheel

inward circles

Swing a wide inward circle with an open hand. You can do this over the front leg or the back leg. The pictures show it over the back leg. That will feel more powerful at first, but you want to get good at both.

"Throw" still means throw! Start big and loose until you get the feel for it.

The flywheel is the most important thing!

Turn your hips and pivot on the ball of your back foot while you make this strike.

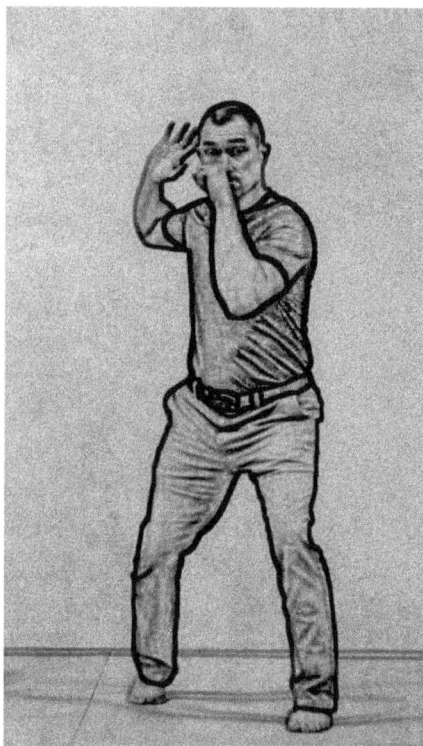

Let your palm hit the focus mitt with a heavy "whap!" Finish the circle by turning your hip and heel to neutral. Return to a compact guard position.

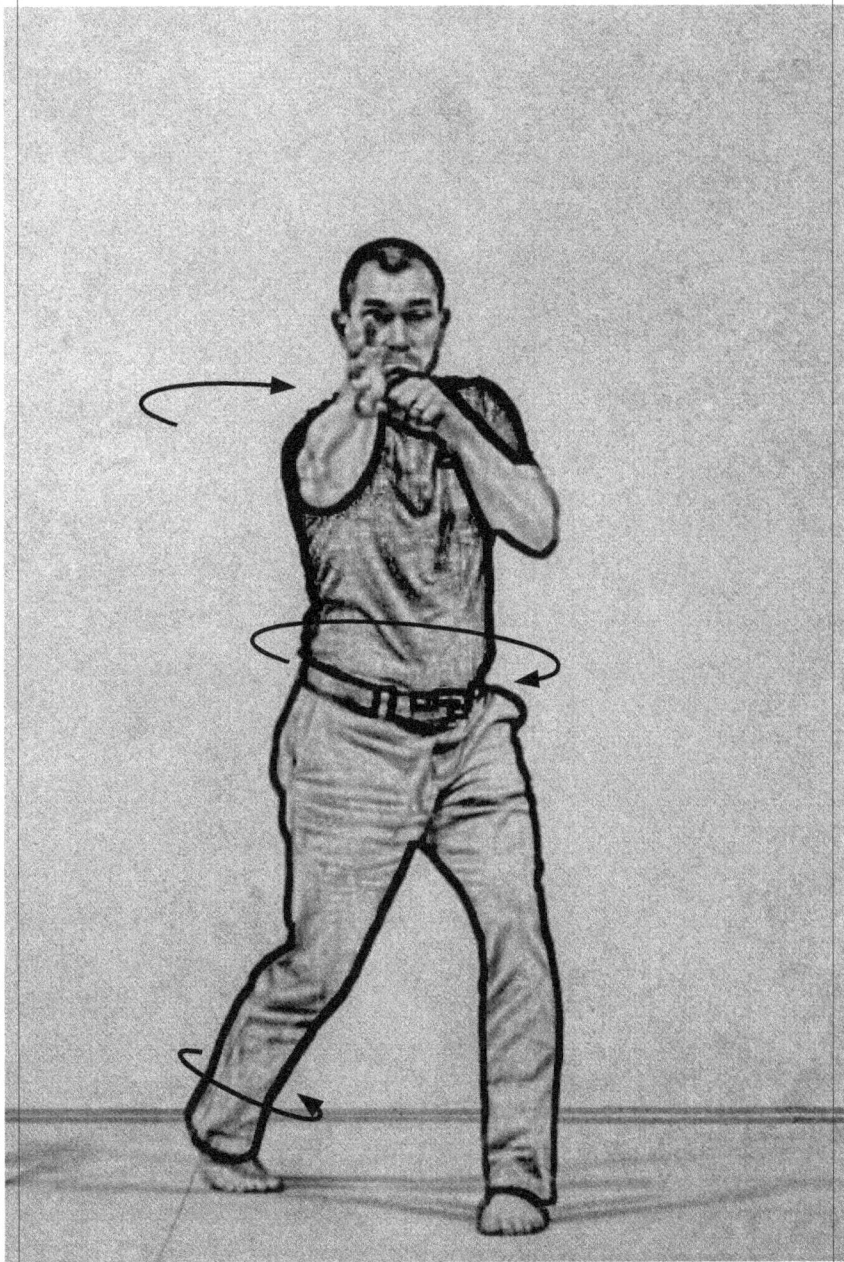

outward circles

Swing a wide outward circle with your hand open, thumb down. It's usually harder to get the feel for this strike than for the inward circle strike. That's why you have to practice more.

You can drag the arm across with your flywheel, or you can use counter-torque.

The pictures show the version where you drag the arm across with the flywheel. To use counter-torque, move the opposite hip back while the arm swings out.

There's a loose shoulder feel that you have to get to really find the power in this strike. Always return to your compact guard position after the strike!

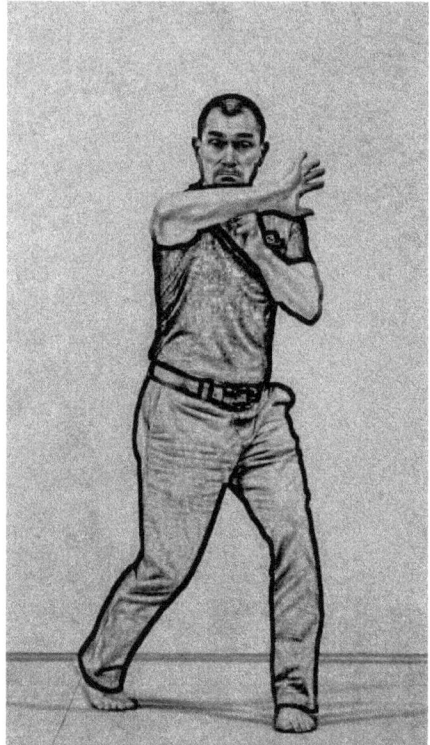

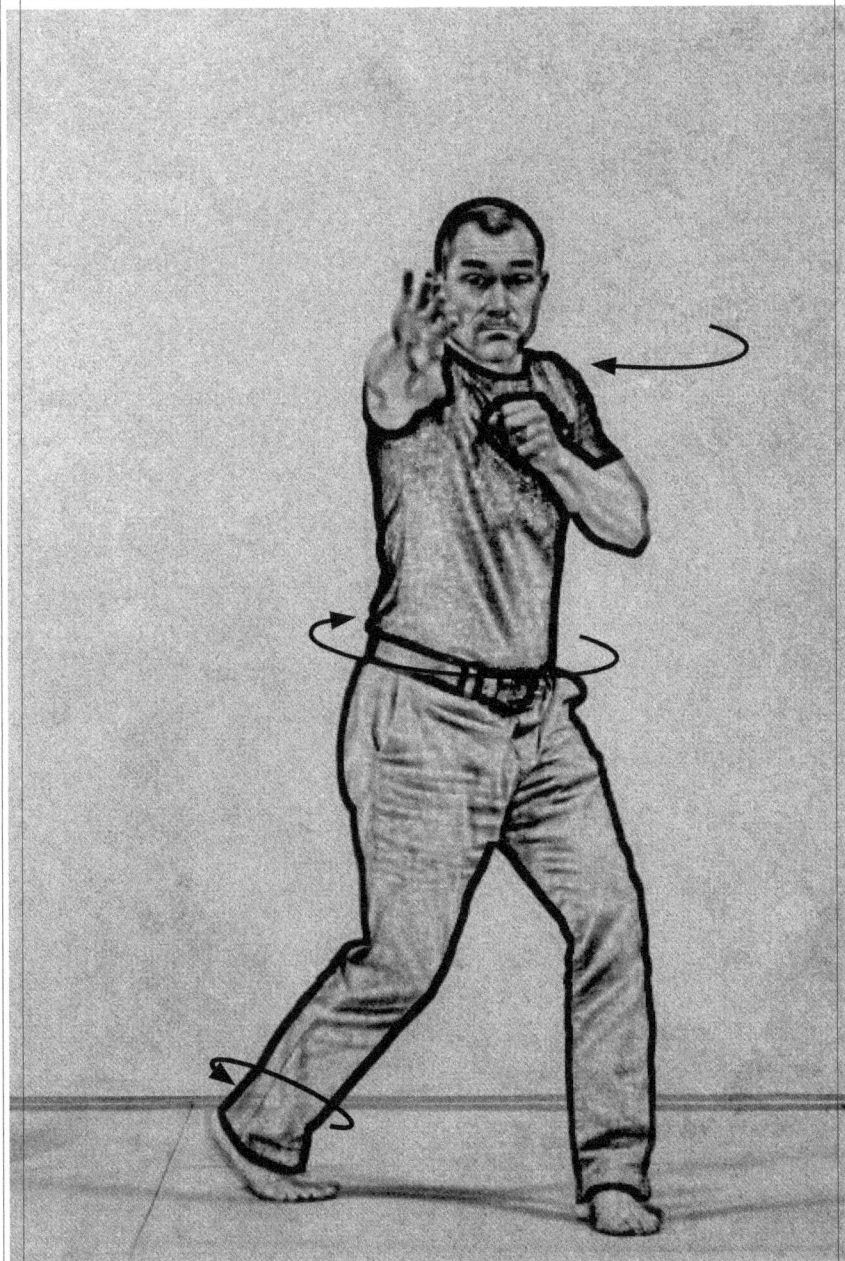

the flywheel

upward circles

This is just like an uppercut with an open hand, but better because only the cool people do it. The power comes from the flywheel. Rotate the flywheel in an upward direction to drive the strike.

Start by dropping the arm behind the hip. The arm passes very close to the side of your body on the way up.

On the opposite page, see how the angles of motion drive power up from the leg? That's true whether you're striking off the back leg or the front leg.

Here's the hard part – the finish position is with the elbow bent, close to your rib cage. This is not an extended arm uppercut. Those are easier to learn but rarely have the sick, heavy power of this strike.

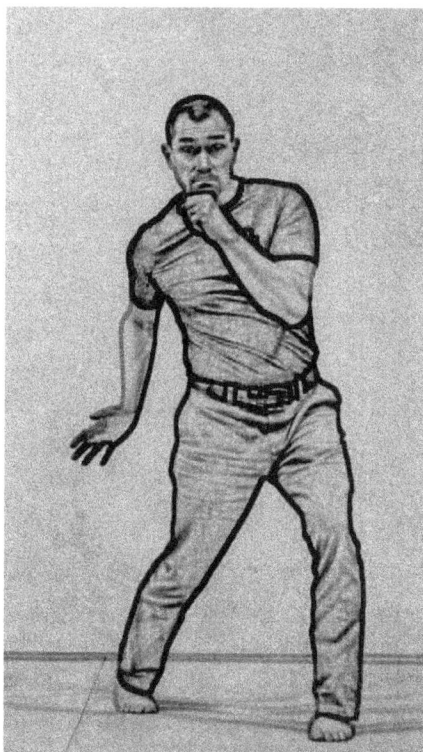

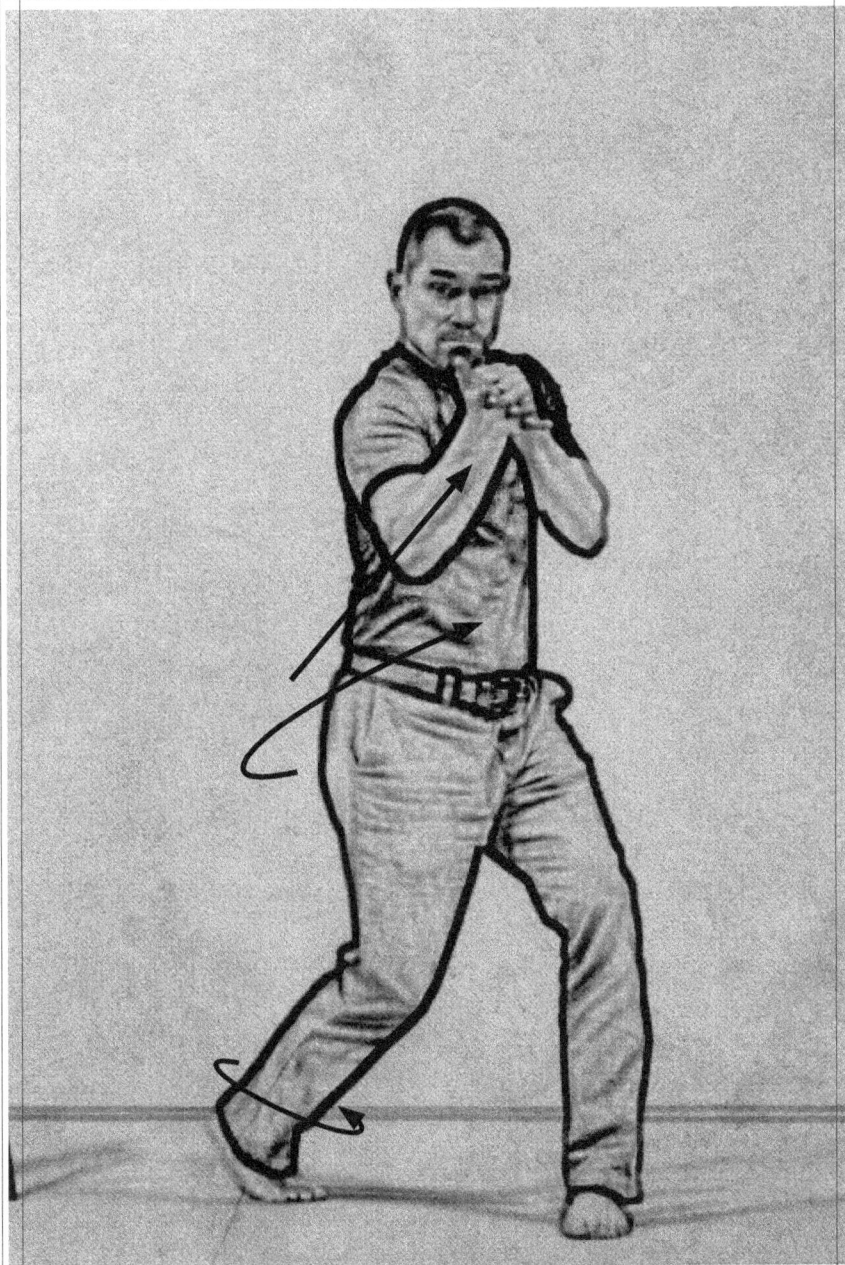

downward circles

This is a heavy downward smash. The power comes from bending the knees and dropping the flywheel as you drop your elbow close to your body.

Lift your hand over your head and drop it on the mitt like a 25lb Olympic weight plate on a fleeing dung beetle.

In practice, you want the mitt at solar plexus height to get the feel for it, but this strike could be used on the bridge of the nose, clavicle, or forearm of an opponent in self-defense. It's a superb part of a mix of strikes in rapid succession.

Practice these open hands strikes singly and in combinations, slow and heavy, fast and light, static and moving, until you can get the same power when you start from the guard postion as you do when you swing wildly.

Always start the flywheel in motion first and keep your hands and arms relaxed.

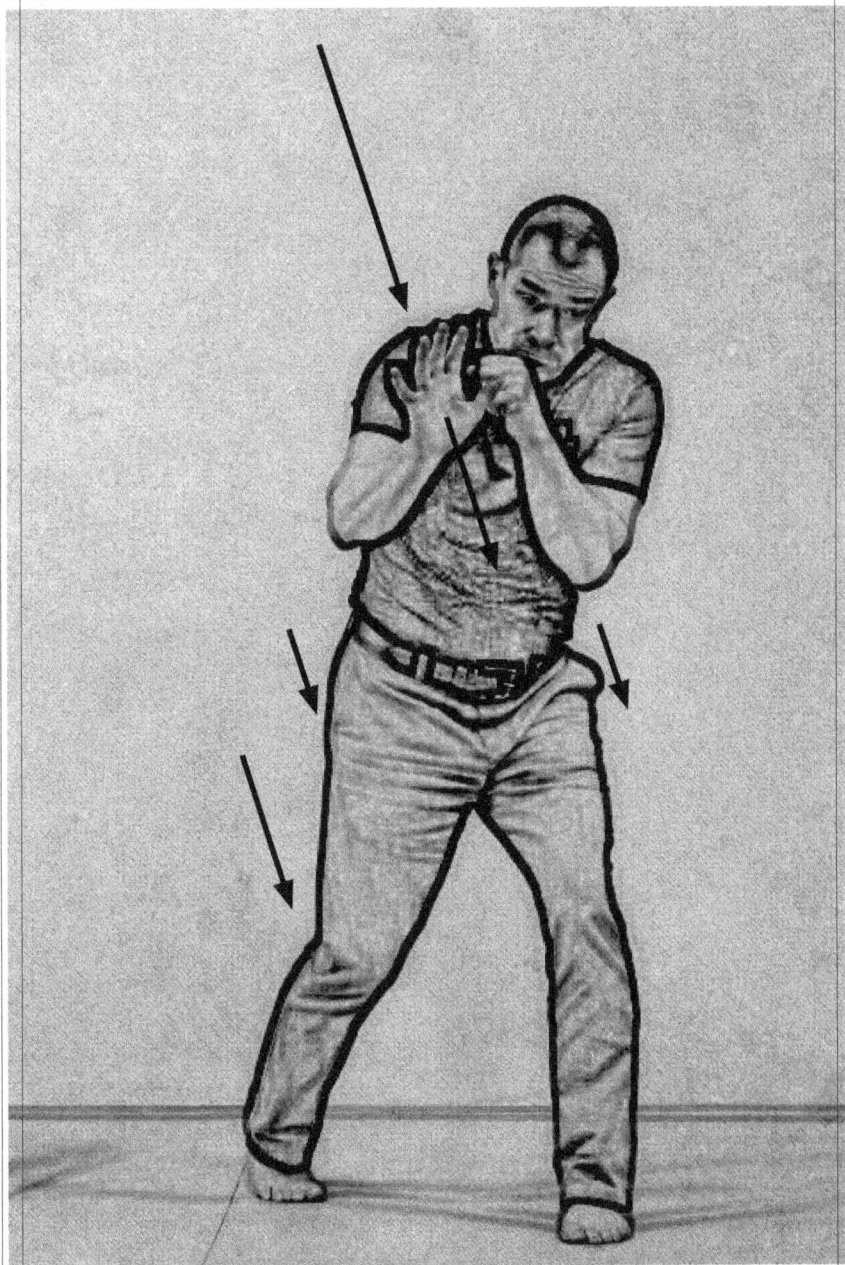

chapter five

fist strikes

"Around every handful of flowers is a clenched fist."
- Uncle Filthy

A fist delivers a more intense power load to the target. It's the *sine qua non* of martial arts tools. Look up the words you don't understand in the dictionary, lasses and laddies!

It takes time to build up a good fist, to condition your knuckles, and to learn to relax your shoulders and arms while you keep your fists tight.

Pay close attention to the lessons, put in the hard work, stay humble, and learn to drop bombs.

Why is "tomb" spelled like "bomb" but not pronounced the same? There's no reason, so stop wasting time and read the next lesson.

the flywheel

how to make a fist

Start with an open hand. Fold your fingers once, then fold them again. Pull the first two fingers tight with your thumb. Hit stuff with the two largest knuckles of the first and second fingers. Line those knuckles up with your forearm bones.

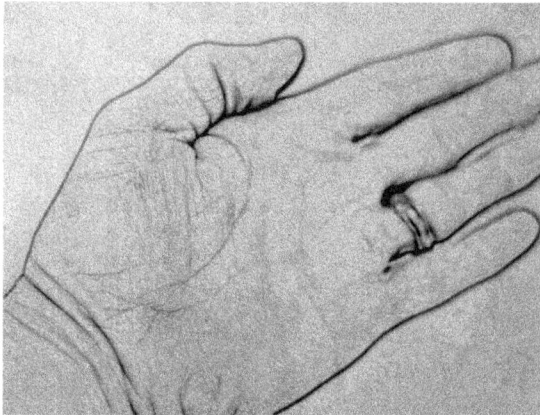

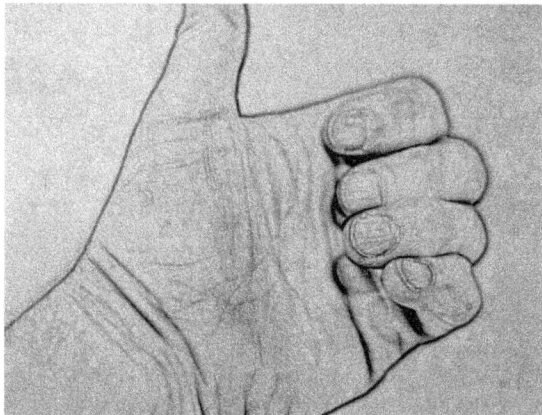

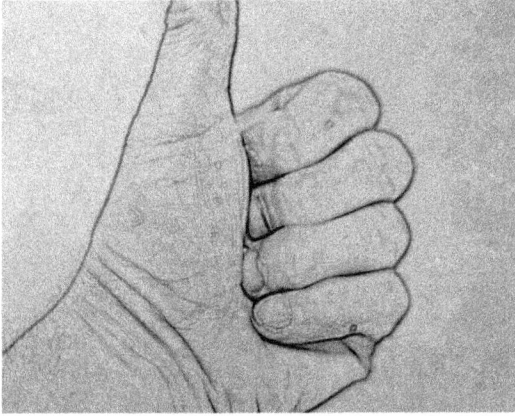

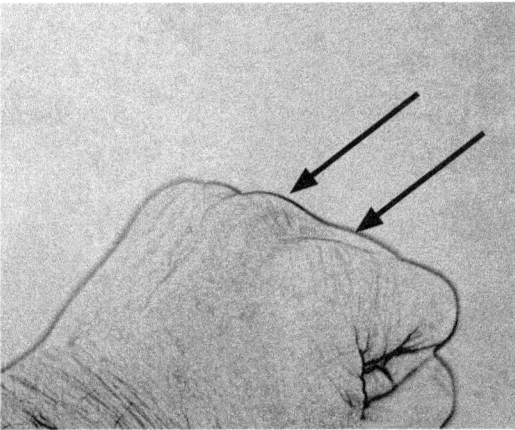

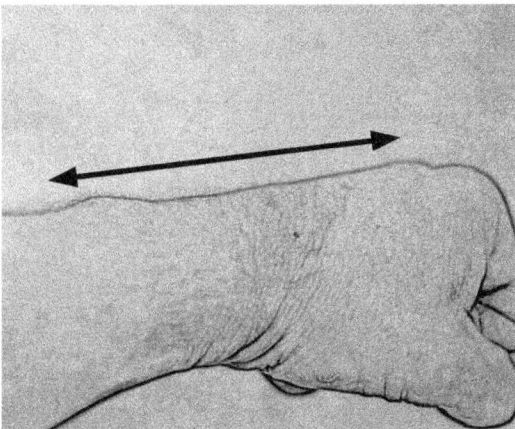

fists tight, shoulders and arms relaxed

To throw fast, powerful punches, you need to be able to keep your fists tight but your arms and shoulders relaxed. Think of your fists like wrecking balls and your arms like chains. The flywheel and the torso provide most of the power – your shoulders and arms are guidance tools, not power tools.

This might take some practice.

Hold your fists in front of you, keeping them tightly clenched. Consciously relax your shoulders and bob them up and down.

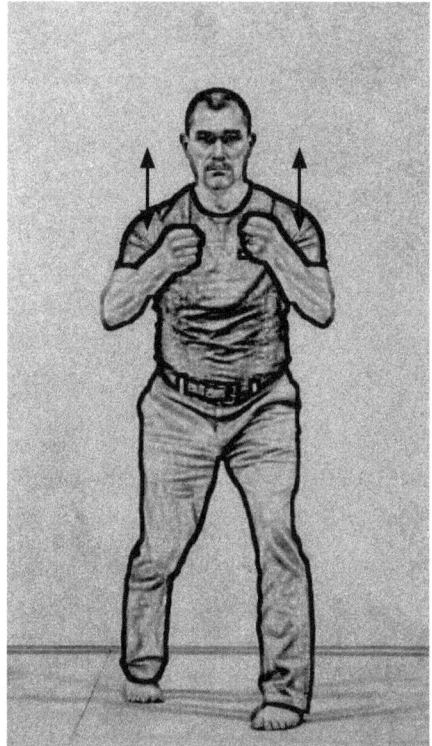

You can also throw your fists around while you keep the rest of your upper body relaxed. Someday you'll look as good doing it as that manly specimen in the pictures.

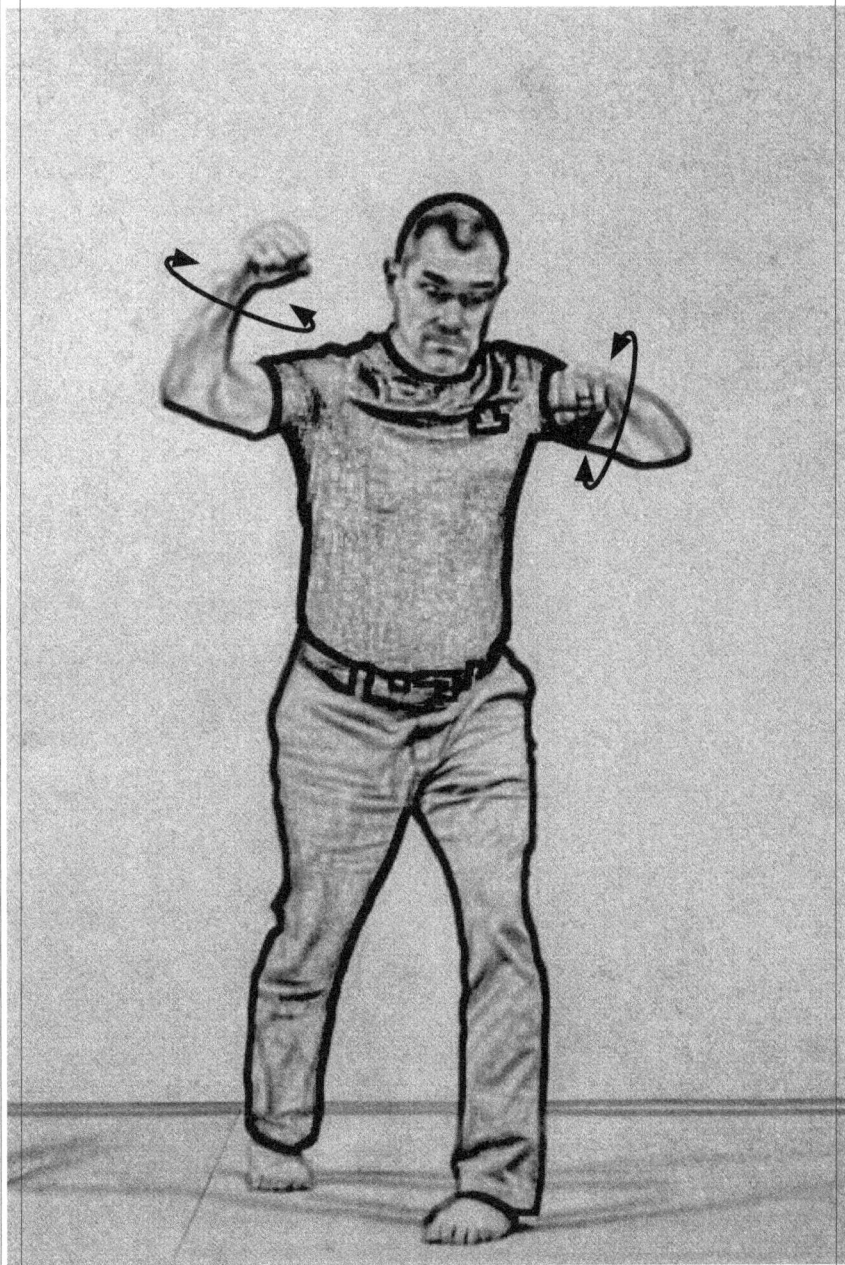

disciplined flywheel jab

Everything about the closed-fist jab is the same as the open hand jab shown earlier, except you throw a fist rather than an open hand. Thank you, Captain Obvious! The power comes from the ball of your back foot and the flywheel. Seek a heavy feeling in the jab. The more relaxed and efficient you are, the heavier it will feel.

Start by pressing the ball of the back foot into the floor. Move the flywheel, then the arm.

Beginners tend to lean into the jab too much. A little lean is okay, a lot is not. Keep your face straight ahead and look at your target the whole time.

Did I mention that you should always return to a relaxed, compact guard position?

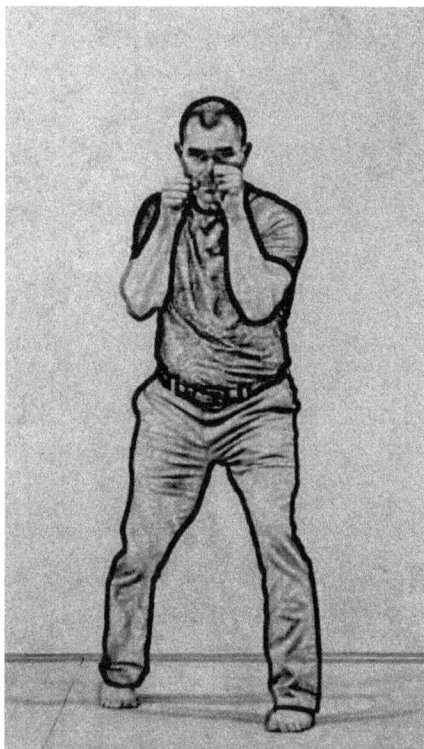

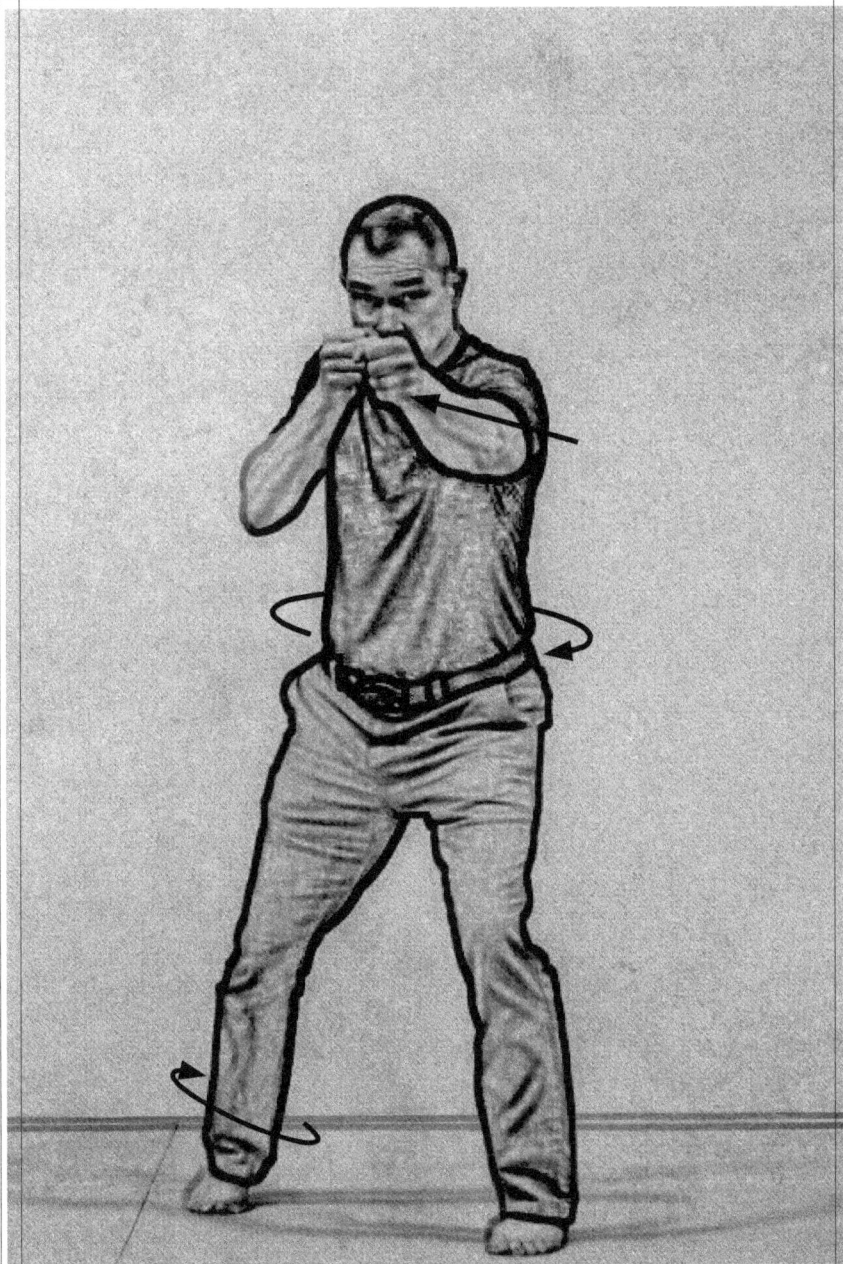

disciplined flywheel cross

The jab comes off the front foot and lead hand, but the cross comes off the back foot and trailing hand. Power, once again, comes from the ball of your back foot and the flywheel. Seek a heavier feeling in the cross than in the jab. Sink into your target. You want your training partner to worry about how hard you're going to hit the focus mitt.

Start the cross by pressing the ball of the back foot into the floor and crouching just a bit. Move the flywheel first, as always, then the arm.

Complete the circle! After the flywheel rotates to drive the punch, it turns back to set you up for the next punch.

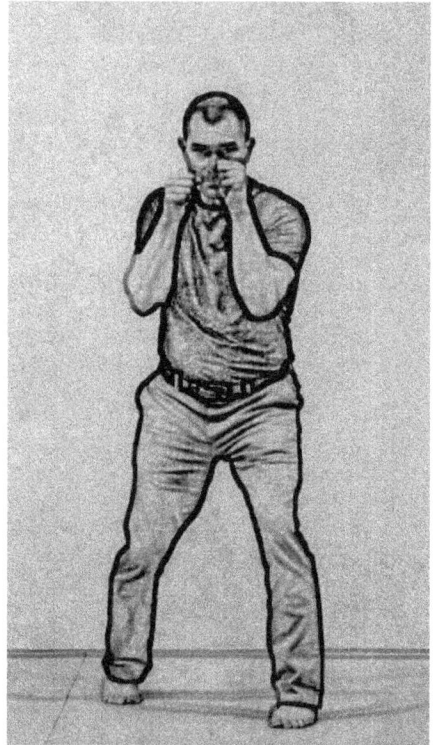

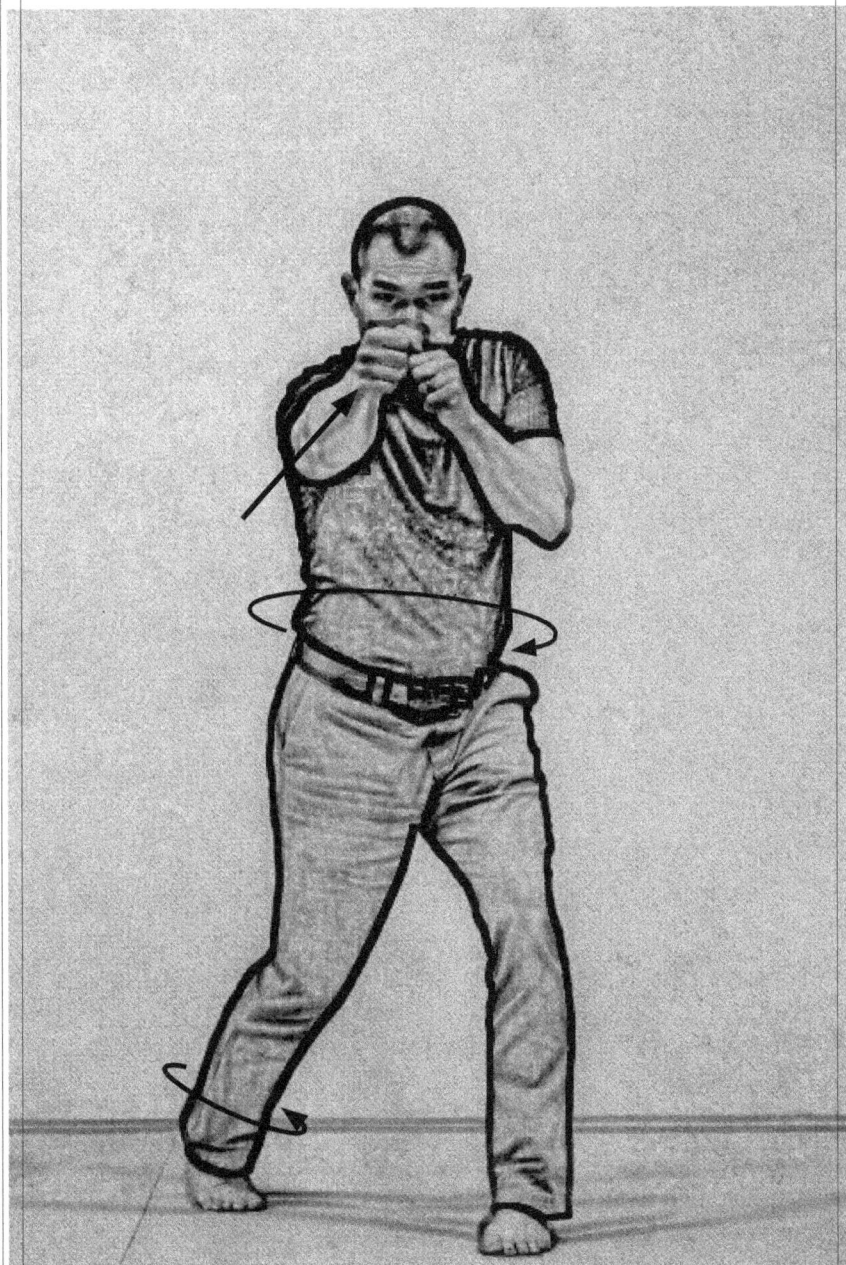

one-two punch

The jab-cross combination. Be sure the hip moves
before the arms move. Always return to a balanced,
relaxed, compact guard position. Drink your milk, take
your vitamins, do your pushups and always wear clean
underwear to the gym.

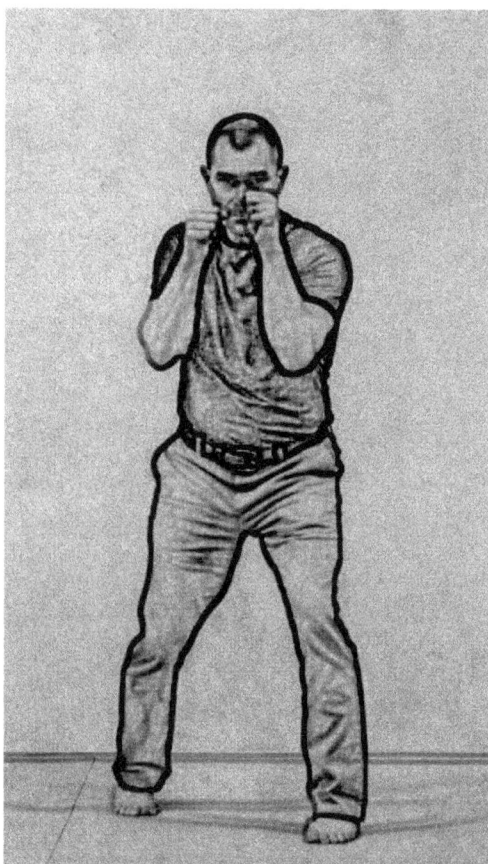

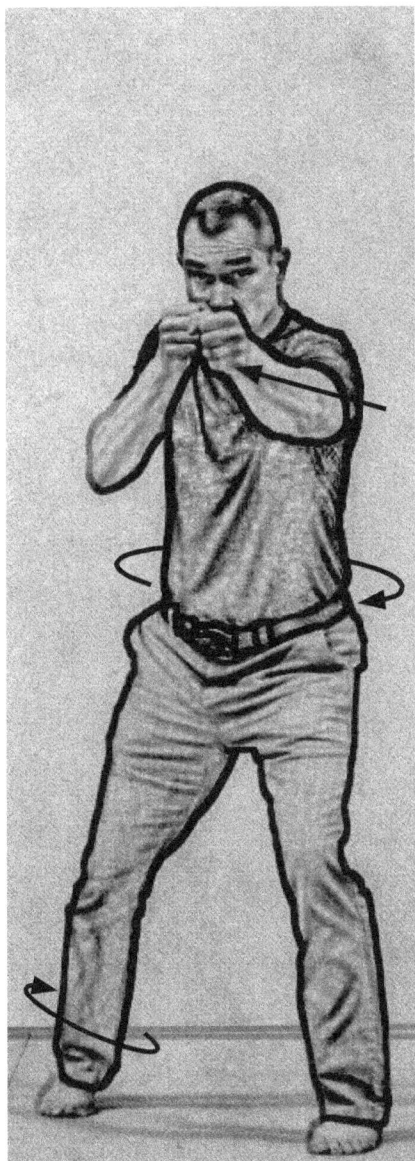
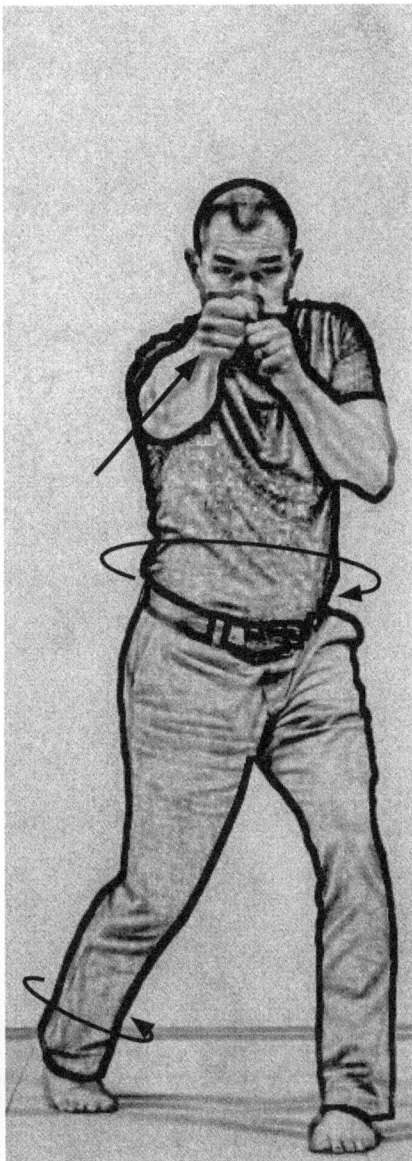

angled uppercut

The angled uppercut comes out of a rotating, rising hip that drives power into the torso and arm. Make it a big motion at first to train the trajectory of the punch. In a few months, you'll be able to generate as much or more power with smaller, more disciplined circles.

The arms travels on an upward angle, with the elbow passing close to the hip.

You can do this strike off the front or back leg, so learn both.

Don't extend the arm to finish the uppercut. Unwind the body instead. There's a sick level of power that comes from connecting your legs, hips, torso, arms and fist in this supreme ice making machine of a finishing punch.

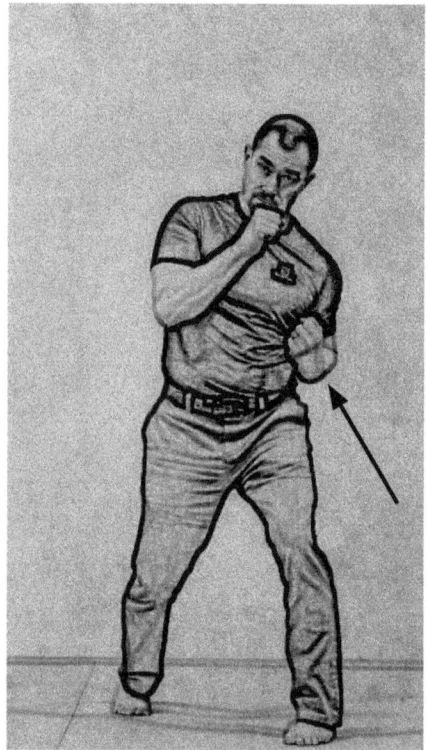

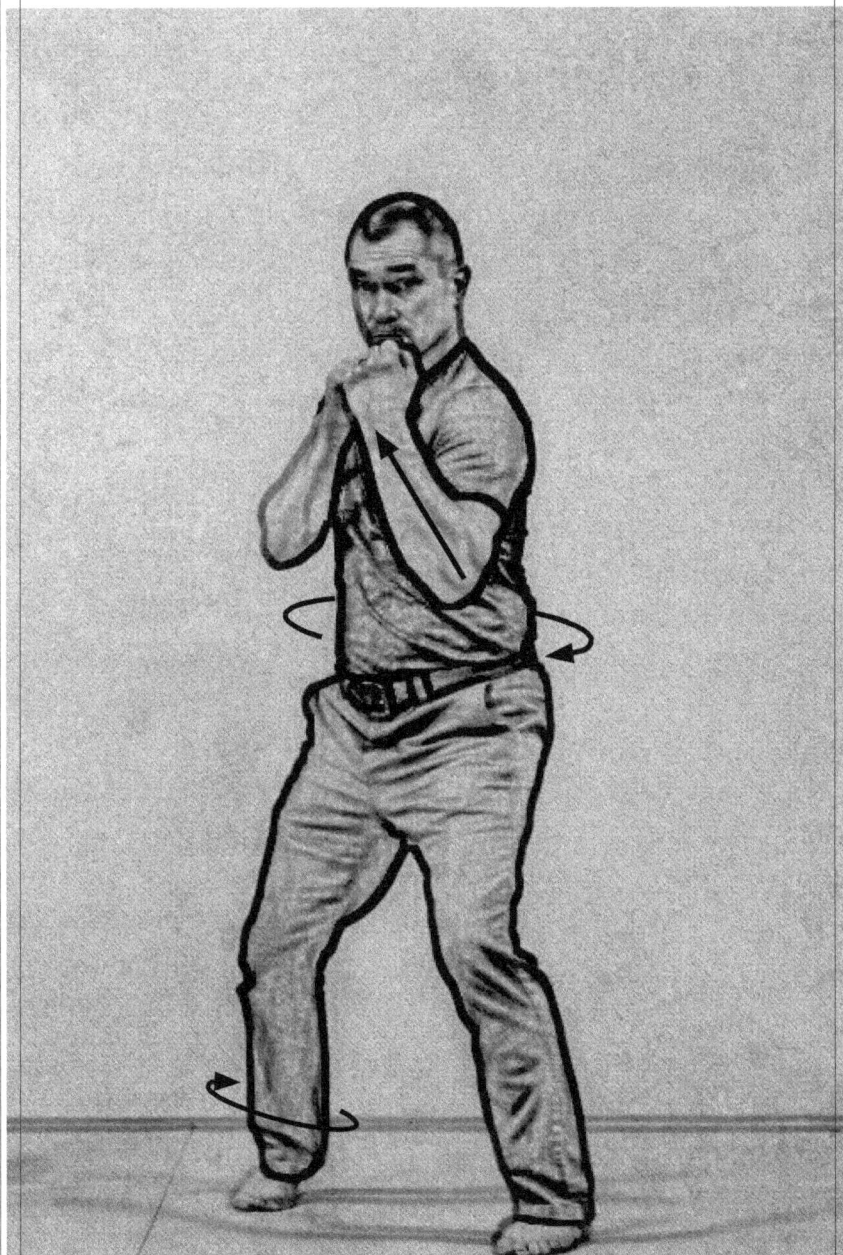

elbow-high hook

The elbow-high hook is a very close-in finishing strike that comes out of the same hip rotation as the jab and inward circle strike. You can fire this off either the front or the back leg, but most of the time the front leg is better. Let the arm drop back, then bring it up into a horizontal circle.

Start with big circles. In a few months, you'll be able to generate as much power with smaller, more disciplined circles.

The finish is palm down, elbow at a right angle, forearm parallel to the floor. Don't extend the arm to finish the strike. Instead, stop the arm and let the momentum of your body finish the heavy strike.

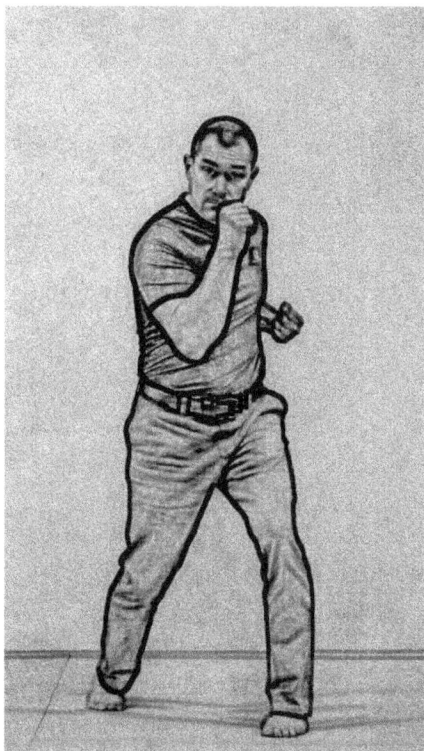

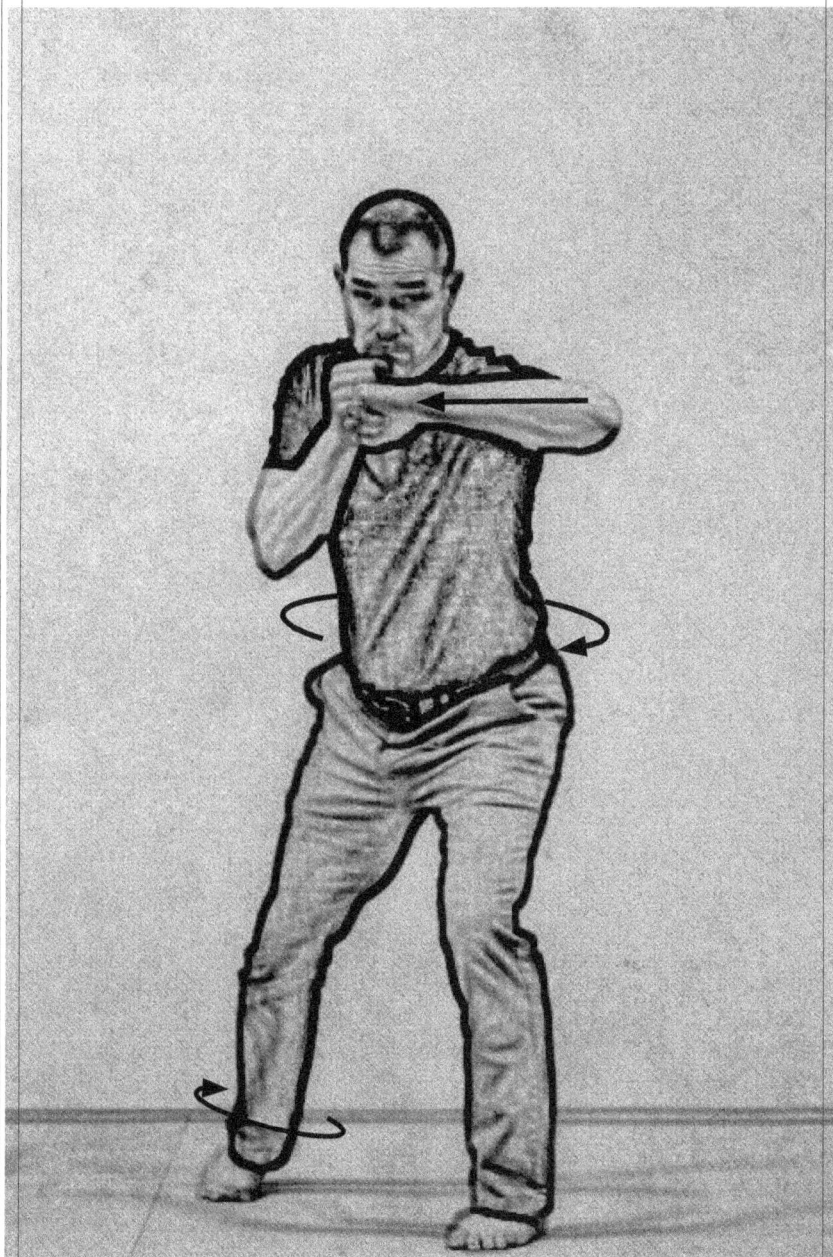

build your skill

Practice stringing together all these closed-fist strikes.
Practice a lot.

- Train solo (shadowboxing) to focus on the hip
  movement and smoothness.
- Train with focus mitts to develop power and reac-
  tive speed.
- Train on the heavy bag to build crushing heaviness and to get your body used to resistance.
- Train with boxing gloves and a partner to learn
  distancing, timing, and tactics.
- Get used to hitting a moving human being and
  getting hit by one.

If you're a couch potato, use big gloves and throw
light strikes until you get in shape.

If you're manly like some of the other meatheads
looking at the pictures in this book, throw heavy
bomb pops, stick and move, and keep your teeth
together. Do I have to tell you everything?

fist strikes
combinations

Here are some combinations to practice (always return to a relaxed, compact guard position):

Jab – cross
Jab – cross – uppercut
Jab – cross – elbow-high hook
Jab – uppercut – cross
Jab – uppercut – elbow-high hook
Jab – cross – uppercut – elbow-high hook
Jab – cross – uppercut – elbow-high hook – cross

Make up a bunch of your own. Try them against a lively partner to see if they hold up. If you get hit in the face a lot, you should rethink your choices.

In the next chapter, we'll add kicks into the mix.

chapter six

kicks

"Maybe what that old dog needs is a good kick in the ass." - Dalai Llama

The hip is the flywheel for kicks, too. For a lot of people, it's harder to get the flywheel into kicks than punches.

To raise your kicking game and get the flywheel moving, you need to learn another ball of the foot move.

Learn to pivot on the ball of the base foot. Practice until you can turn the base foot 180-degrees so that the heel points at the target.

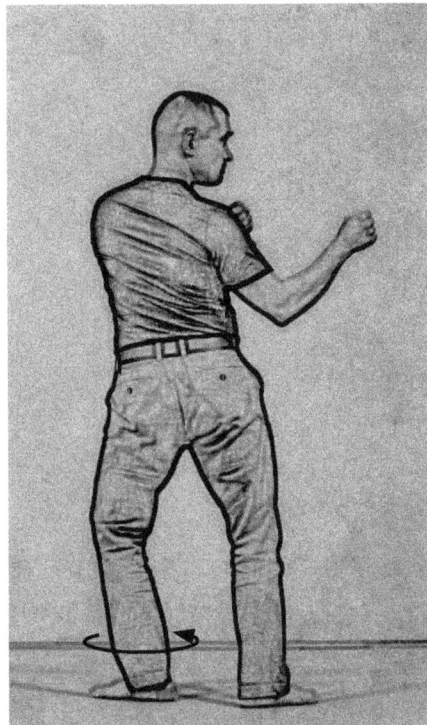

the hip is the flywheel

Notice how pivoting on the ball of the foot lets you swing your hip toward the target.

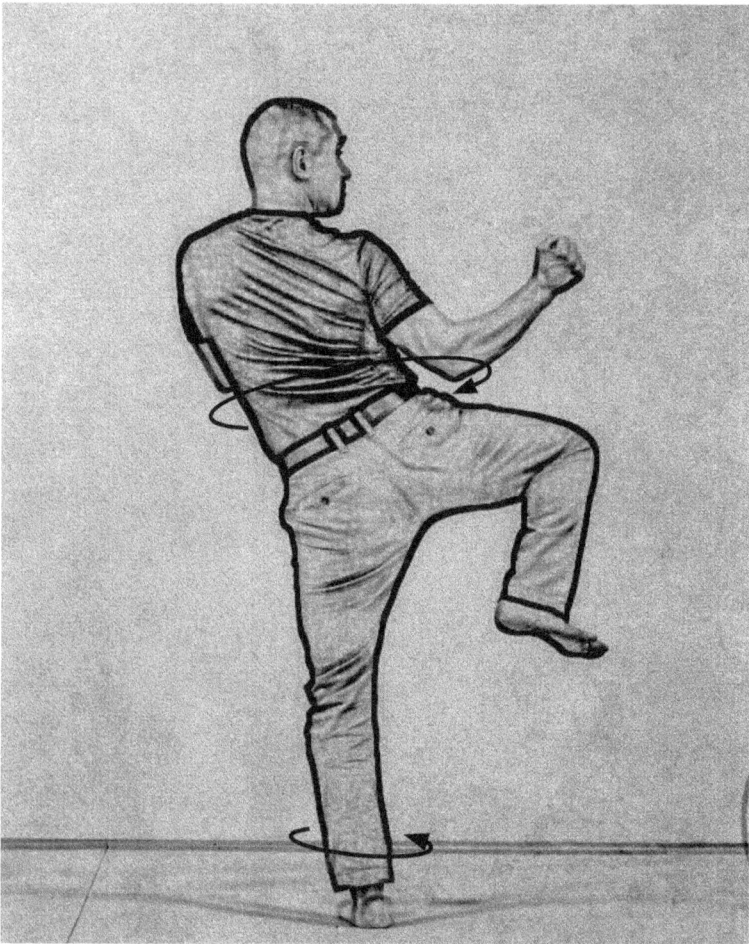

free up the kicking leg

Your legs have to be able to move fluidly. Practice pivoting on the ball of your foot, letting your hip swing around, and pointing your lead knee at the target.

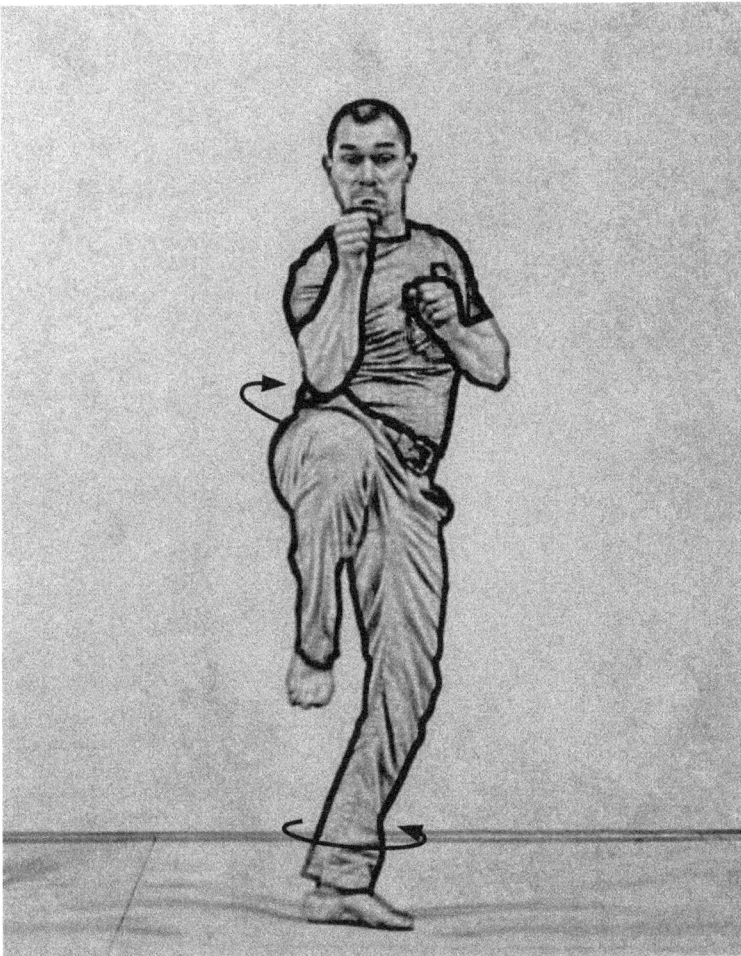

the flywheel

back-leg front kicks

Learn the back leg version of the kicks first. It's bigger, easier and you can get more power. When you have a good feeling for the back leg version, start working on the front leg version.

Turn the base foot out to start the hip forward. Let the hip swing forward to drive the kicking knee toward the target.

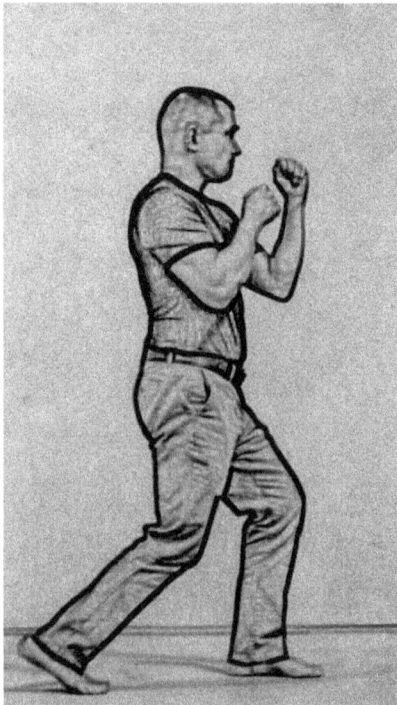

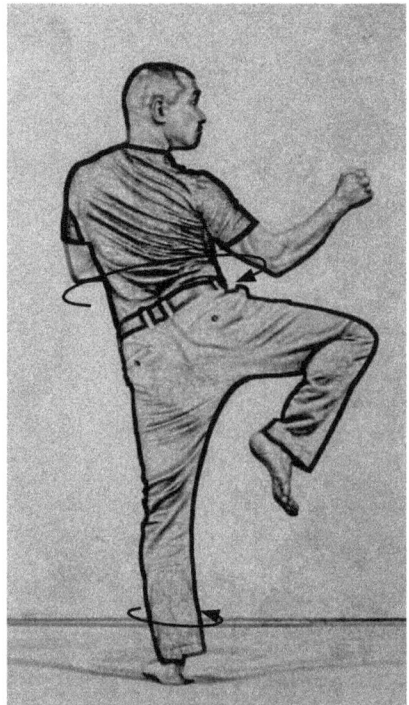

front-leg front kicks

Step slightly forward with the back leg to set up the pivot point. Make a small circle with the flywheel to start the kicking knee forward. Drive hard off the ball of the back foot to create linear power. You can do quick snap kicks or drive hard through your target like the love-muffin in the picture below.

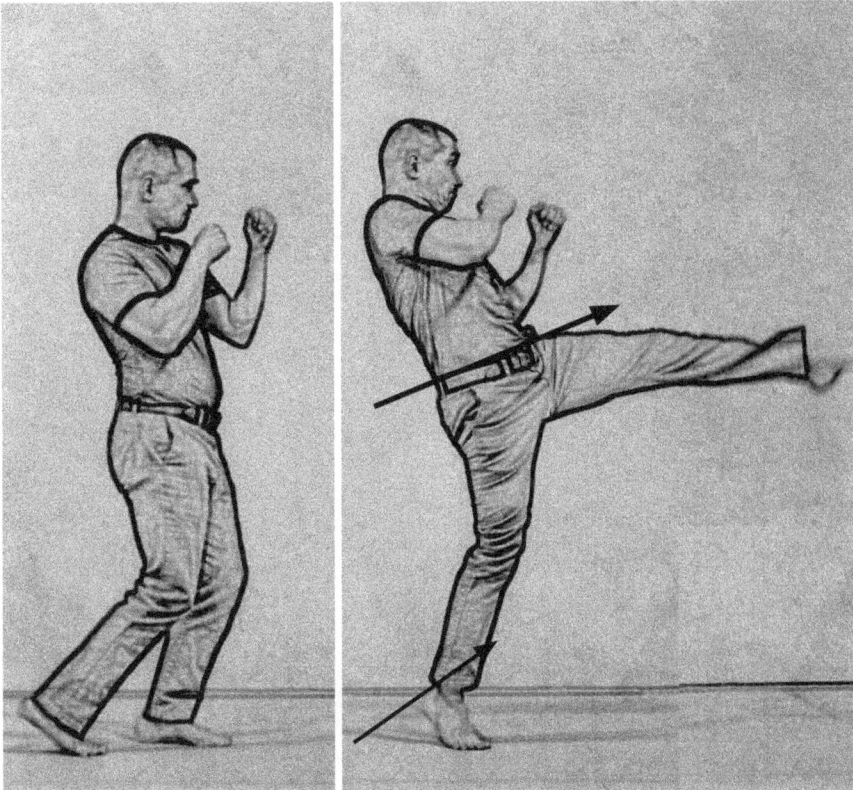

back-leg round kicks

Turn the base foot out to start the hip forward. Let the hip swing forward to drive the kicking knee toward the target. Turn your leg over and extend to drive the instep or ball of the foot into the target.

You can do a full, raised-knee round kick or bring it up quick with foot and hip rotation as shown in the photo below.

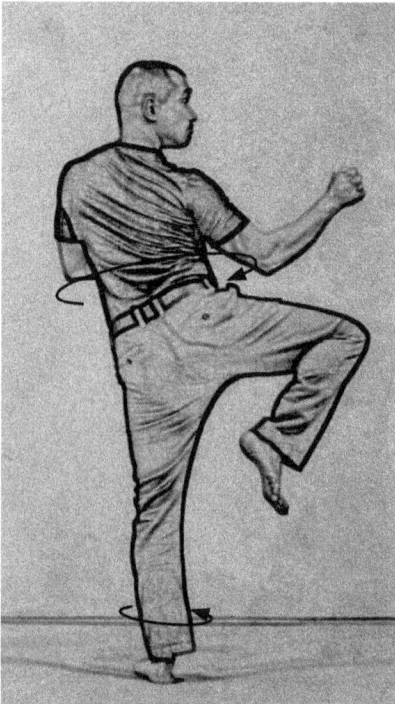

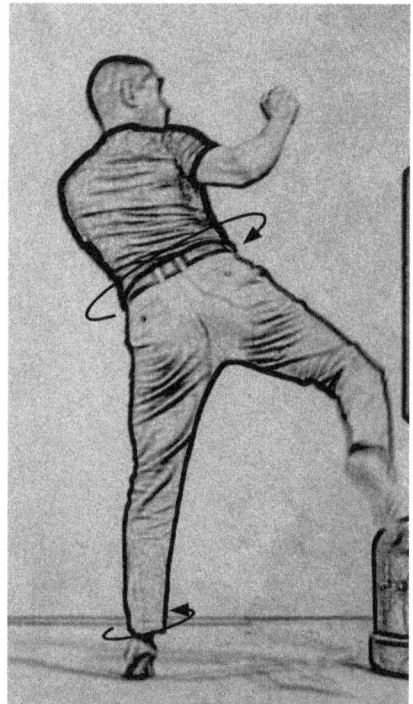

front-leg round kicks

Step slightly forward with the back leg to set the pivot
point. Make a small circle with the flywheel to start the
kicking knee forward. Turn your leg over and extend to
drive the instep or ball of the foot into the target. Vary
the amount of pivot depending on distance and how
committed you are to the kick.

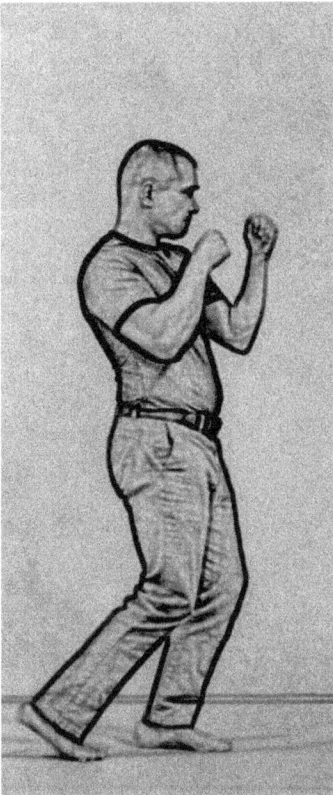

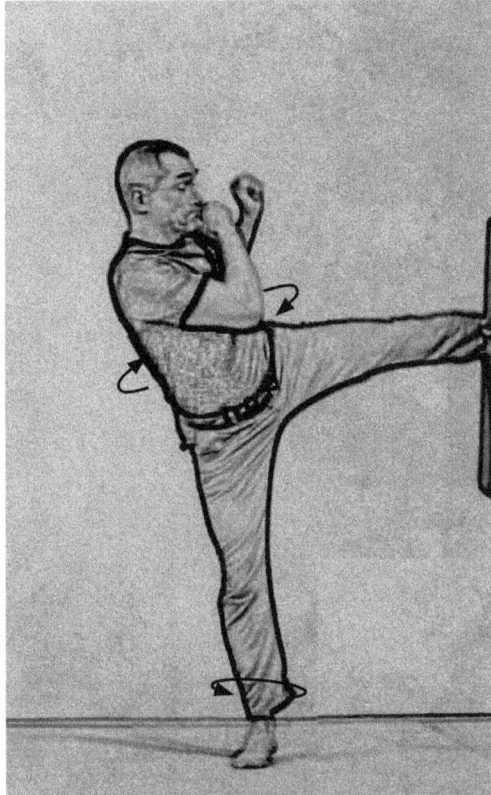

the flywheel

back-leg side kicks

Turn the base foot out to start the hip forward. Let the hip swing forward to drive the kicking knee toward the target. Turn the hip over and extend the leg to drive your heel into the target. Open your hips and get good extention – it's all connected.

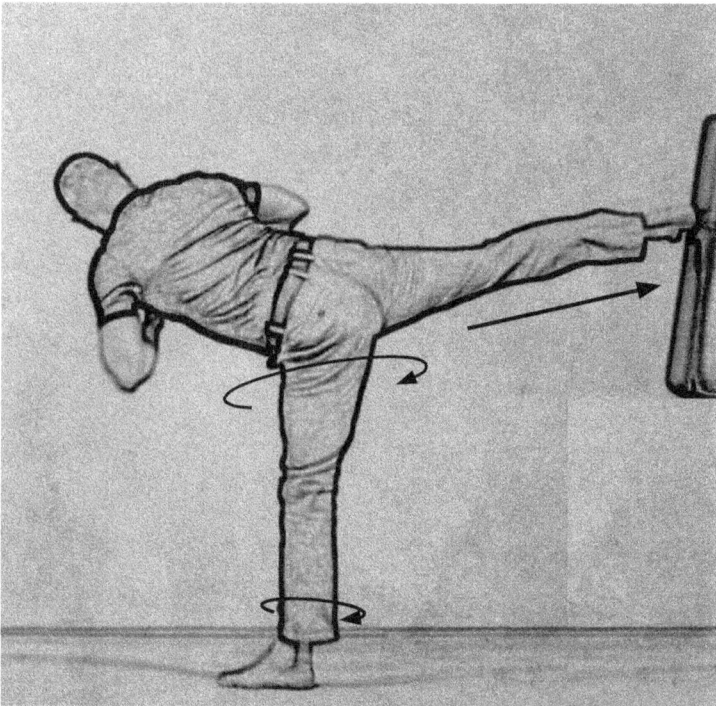

front-leg side kicks

Step slightly forward with the back leg to set up the pivot point. Make a small circle with the flywheel to start the kicking knee forward. Turn the hip over and extend the leg to drive your heel into the target.

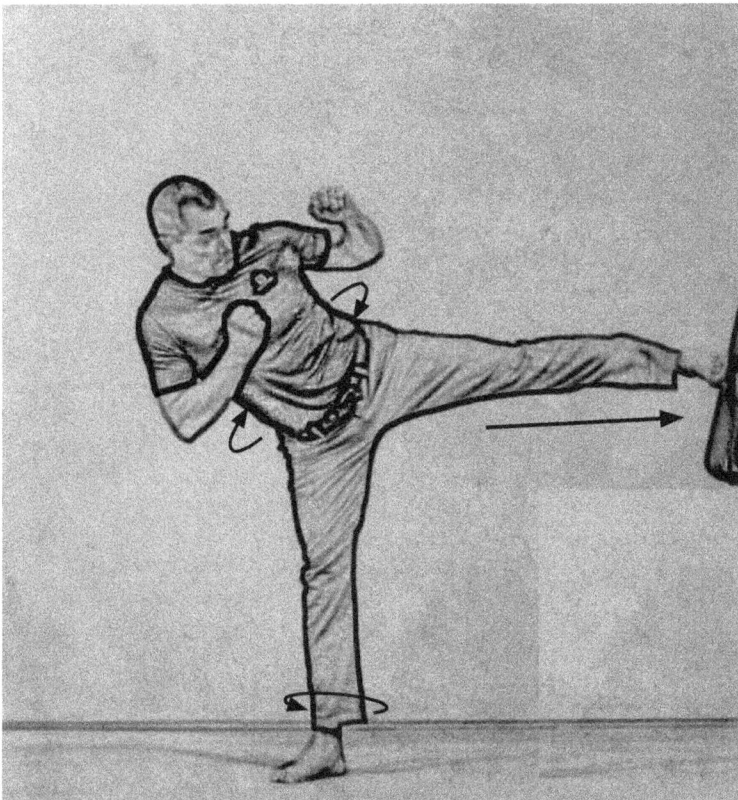

chapter seven

power multipliers

"Less isn't more. More is more."
- Madeleine Albright

There are many ways to strike harder. The quickest way is to add more effort, but that leads to tighter muscles, less accuracy, more fatigue, and more difficulty getting back to a compact, relaxed guard position.

Use the flywheel. Strive to add power while staying relaxed, in balance and preserving your ability return to a compact guard, ready to move.

Some better ways to multiply your power within the flywheel system are:

1. get better at turning your hips;
2. get better at pushing off with the ball of your foot;
3. step forward;
4. step to the side; and
5. add load to your supporting leg.

power generator #1

As you "A" students have figured out, one of our two primary power generators is the flywheel. Turn it at the right time, at the right speed, with the right amount of force. That's the set of subtle skills you need to develop.

Practice every reasonable way you can think of so your punches and kicks get stronger without a lot more muscular effort. Try these:

- Stretching.
- Yoga.
- Hip trainers.
- Resistance bands.
- Salsa dancing.

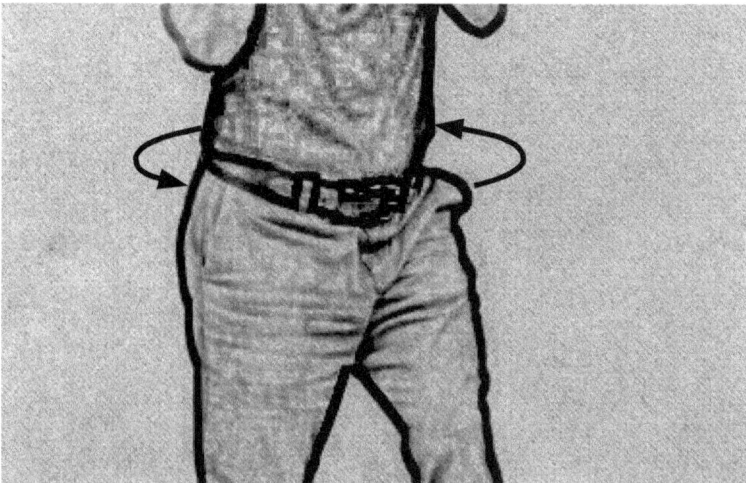

power generator #2

The other primary power generator is the ball of the foot. Transmit maximum force from the floor, through your body and into the target.

Try these things:

- Calf raises with weight.
- Pushing off the floor with the ball of your foot.
- Balancing on the ball of one foot.
- Practicing in front of a mirror in a tutu
- Singing camp songs with a puppy.

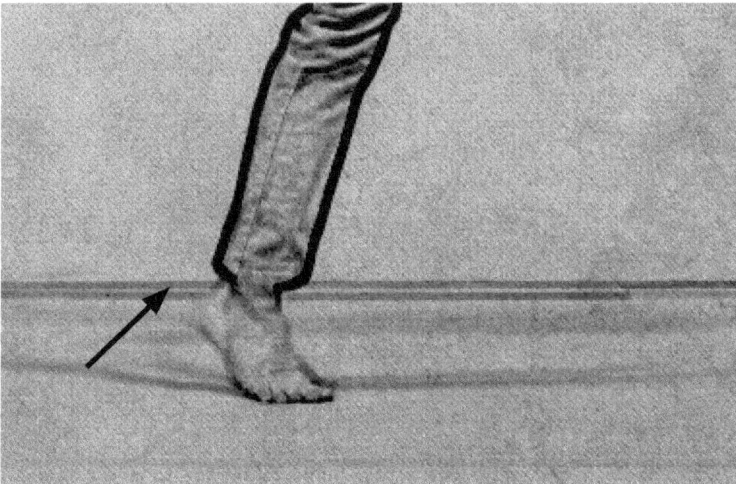

multiply by stepping forward

Push off the ball of the back foot, then pull your back foot forward to the power position. Practice using the push to drive power all the way into the jab, then return to your compact ready position.

Once the step-in jab feels good, practice throwing the cross as soon as your back foot lands in the power position. The key driver for this whole system is hip rotation, so don't lose that when you step forward for extra power.

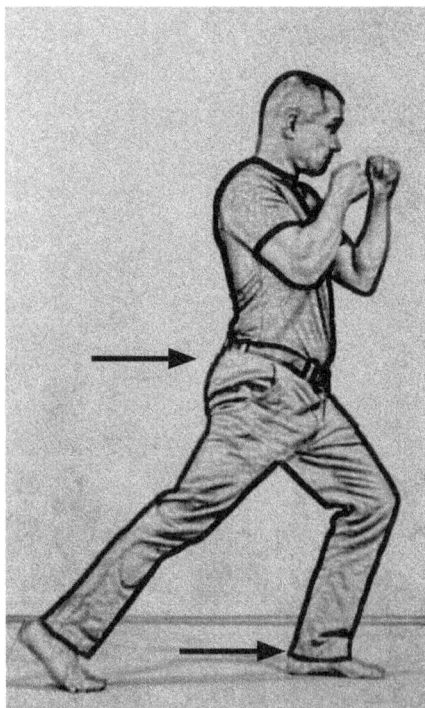

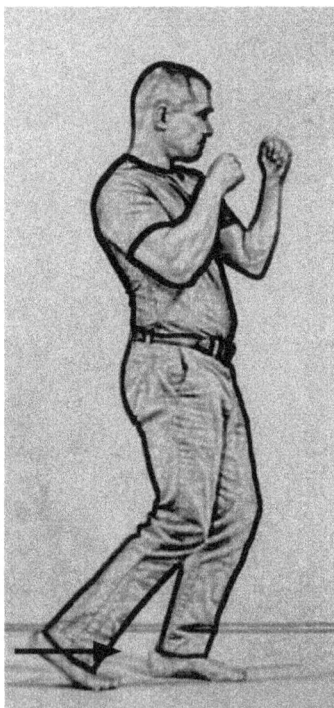

multiply by stepping to the side

Step to the side to load the base leg and open your hips. Your follow-up strike will be pre-loaded for extra power.

Stepping to the side helps build tactical position, too. You can step out of the way of an attack and get useful angles. On the left below, the upper body is canted to avoid the attack before the missle gets launched.

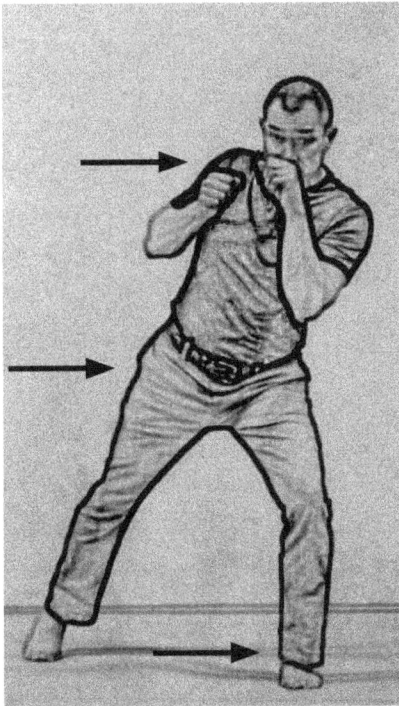

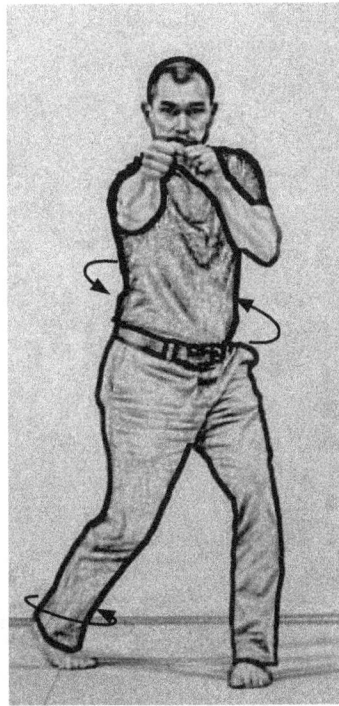

the flywheel

multiply by bending your knees

Your legs are powerful. Well, they would be if you ate a
decent diet and got off the couch once in awhile. Use
them to get more power into your strikes. Move with
more knee bend, then unleash the energy with great fury.

Uncorking bent knees can help with linear power delivery or with rotational power through the flywheel. This
set of pictures shows how you can double up power
sources by combining leg power with flywheel power.

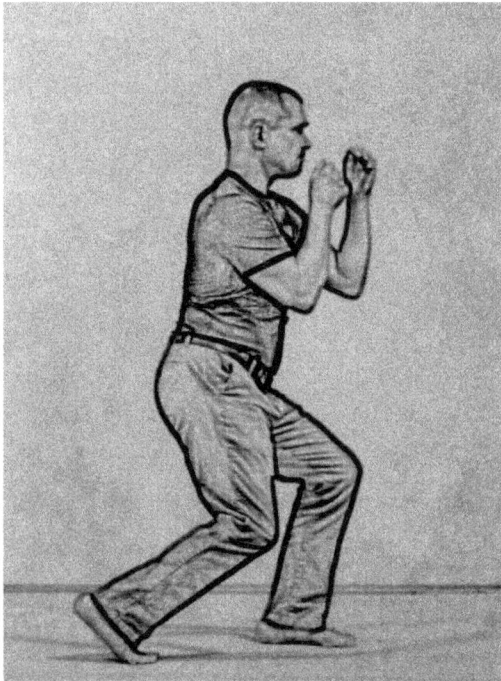

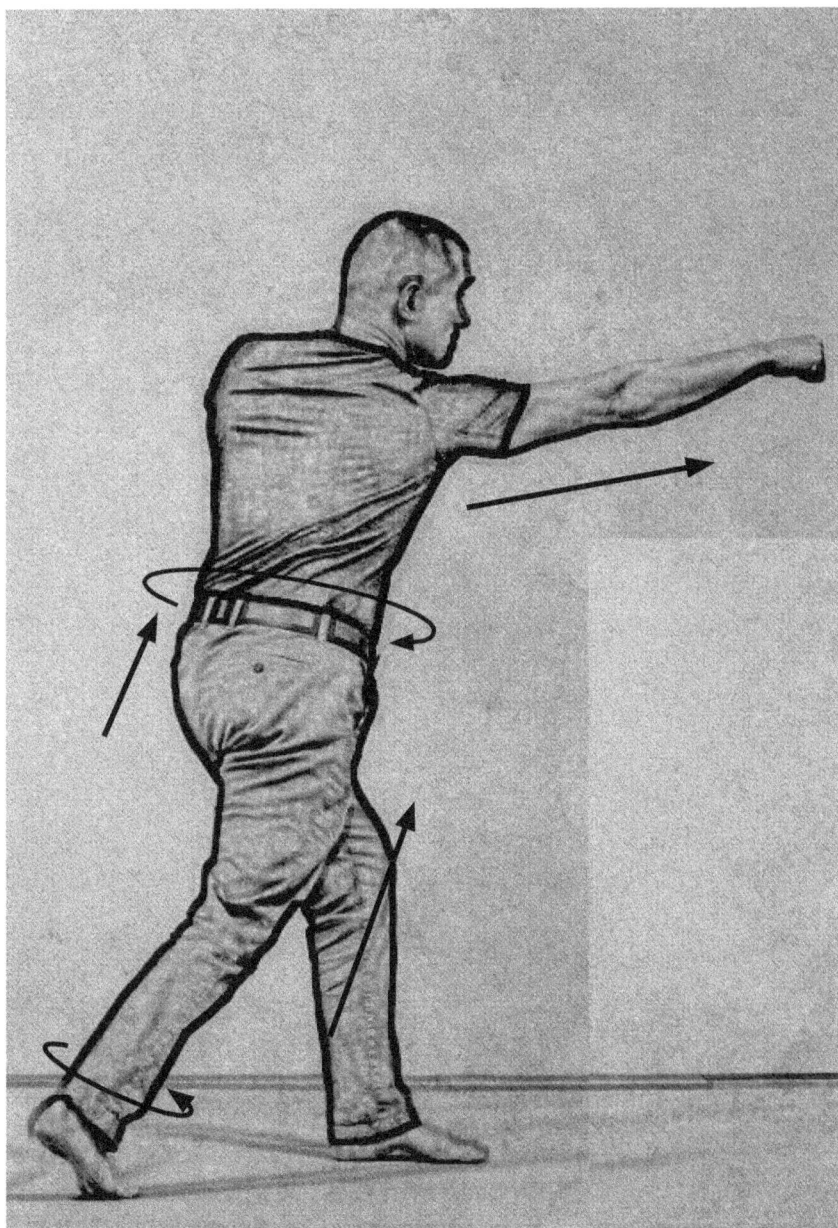

the flywheel

what's next?

**"The thing that comes after this thing?
That's the next thing."
- Deng Xiao Ping**

Practice stringing together all your moves – open hand strikes, punches and kicks. Build effective and intelligent combinations that take advantage of the continuous power delivery of the flywheel.

Typically entering with a jab or front-leg front kick works best because those moves are quicker and less committed than the big bombs like rear-leg front kicks and cross or reverse punches. So the lead-in moves are good places to start your combinations.

But your thing may be a big round kick to start your flow. So be it. Make that work for you, just don't delude yourself about how effective it really is.

That's one of the big problems with a lot of martial arts practice these days... no pressure testing. You need real human beings pushing you to see how your stuff holds up. At the same time, all fighting and no form will cause you to reach your innate limits and not go much further.

the flywheel

To really grow in the combative arts, you need time to practice the basics, you need thoughtful practice of complex movements, and you need pressure testing.

• • •

This book is only an introduction to core principles of the flywheel system. There is a complete methodology of movements and applications that can add power, freedom of movement and creativity to almost every form of hand-to-hand combative art.

You can find more information about *The Flywheel* System at:

https://nicklaus-suino.com/flywheel/the-flywheel-system

what's next?

about doc spears

John "Doc" Spears is a weapons and tactics instructor, spine surgeon, and science fiction writer.

Learn more about his work at:
https://forgetactical.com

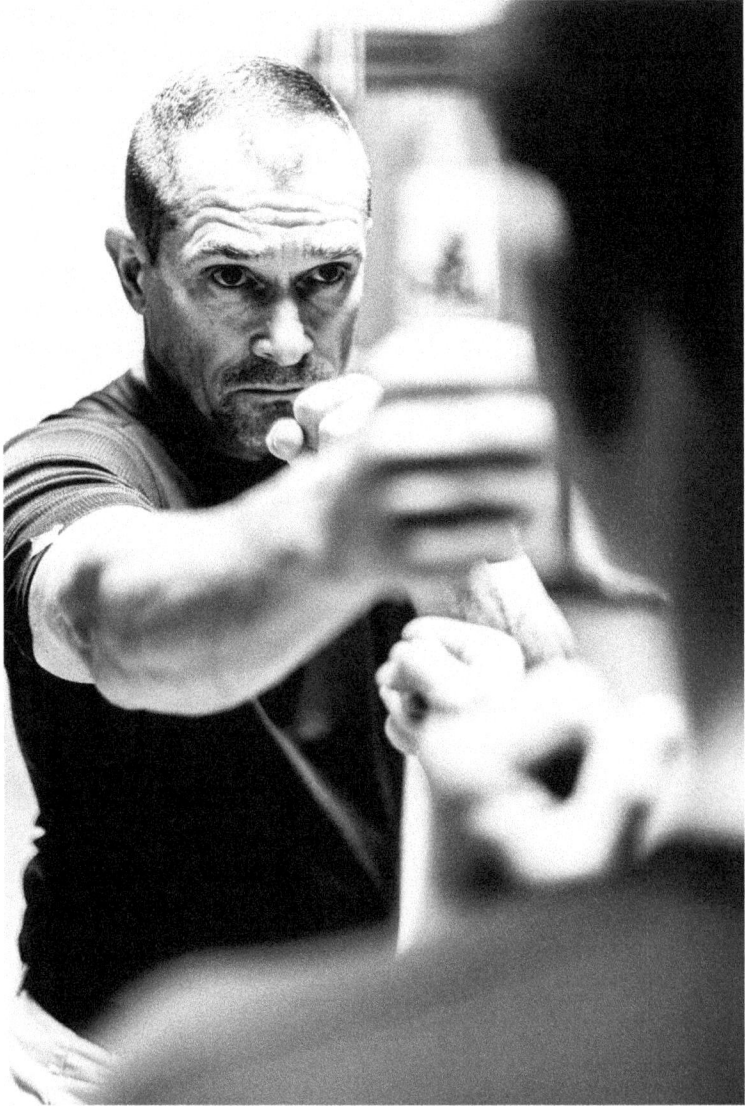

meet the author

For over three decades, thousands of people have become more centered, happier, and more successful with Nick's guidance. He has been called "one of the leading martial arts instructors in North America," but his influence radiates far beyond the dojo. He has made it his life's mission to learn the fundamental principles of success in many different fields, apply them, and share them with people.

Author of many books, including *Look Up!* and *Budo Mind and Body* (named "Essential Gear" by Black Belt Magazine), Nick has helped transform professionals, business owners, athletes, martial artists, and ordinary people with his presentations, group training and coaching. His book *Practice Drills for Japanese Swordsmanship* spent many weeks as the #1 selling title in the Fencing Books category on Amazon.

Nick owns all or part of successful businesses in diverse fields like martial arts, marketing, publishing and law. He has been honored by the University of Michigan–Dearborn as "Mentor of the Year"; by the Bluewater

Chamber of Commerce's Business Expo for advancing entrepreneurship; and by the International Martial Arts Federation for supporting traditional Japanese budo. He and his work have been featured in a wide range of publications, including Black Belt Magazine, The ANN Magazine, and the Journal of Asian Martial Arts.

He's taught self-defense and empowerment to hundreds of men, women, girls and boys. Nick and his teams have a commitment to support worthwhile causes – it's an essential part of their mission. They've donated to dozens of organizations in the past decade, including Fisher House of Michigan, Boy Scouts of America, Alzheimer's Association, SafeHouse of Ann Arbor, Center for Independent Living, and Wounded Warrior Project. See what Nick's up to now at:

https://nicklaus-suino.com/

Sorry-ass technique photos by Nicklaus Suino

Cover and profile photos by Hassan Hodges
See more of his exceptional work at:
https://www.hassanhodgesphotography.com

www.ingramcontent.com/pod-product-compliance
Lightning Source LLC
Chambersburg PA
CBHW030845090426
42737CB00009B/1114